GUIDE BOOK FOR
RETAIL AND WHOLESALE PHARMACY

Sunny Sinha
(M.Pharm)

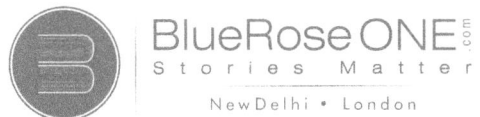

BLUEROSE PUBLISHERS
India | U.K.

Copyright © Sunny Sinha 2024

All rights reserved by author. No part of this publication may be reproduced, stored in a retrieval system or transmitted in any form or by any means, electronic, mechanical, photocopying, recording or otherwise, without the prior permission of the author. Although every precaution has been taken to verify the accuracy of the information contained herein, the publisher assumes no responsibility for any errors or omissions. No liability is assumed for damages that may result from the use of information contained within.

BlueRose Publishers takes no responsibility for any damages, losses, or liabilities that may arise from the use or misuse of the information, products, or services provided in this publication.

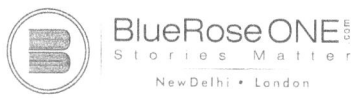

For permissions requests or inquiries regarding this publication, please contact:

BLUEROSE PUBLISHERS
www.BlueRoseONE.com
info@bluerosepublishers.com
+91 8882 898 898
+4407342408967

ISBN: 978-93-6261-660-9

Cover design: Shivam
Typesetting: Namrata Saini

First Edition: July 2024

Preface

In 2015, when I completed my Master in Pharmacy (Pharmacology) it was always in my mind to make the law of the land related to Drugs and Medical Devices (i.e. Drugs and Cosmetics Act and Rules) easily understandable by Indian Pharmacies and Pharmacists who are involved in the business of Drugs and Medical Devices in India. Since, Pharmacists are the custodian of the dispensing of safe drugs to the patient they should be able to understand the laws related to the sale, stock and distribution of Drugs and Medical Devices. In recent years, the Government of India has brought many changes related to the Drugs and Medical Devices Rules, hence it becomes difficult for pharmacists and pharmacies owners to interpret regulatory compliance required to be followed related to the sale, stock and distribution of drugs and medical devices. To fill this gap, I have reviewed a wide variety of topics on the Drugs and Cosmetics Act and Rules thereby extracting out the vital points which a pharmacy needs to follow for the Drugs and Medical devices business. It will be useful and act as a guide book for both online and offline pharmacies in India.

At last but not least, I hope no infringement of Copyrights has been done in this publication and this book would be considered to be one of the valuable resource to all the pharmacies and pharmacists including medical devices bussiness owner for the sake of knowledge gain related to sale, stock and distrbituion of the drugs and medical devices in India.

On 2 Nov 2023, I completed 38 years of my life with the blessings of Lord Shiva and Maa Parvati Adi Shakti. I would like to thank my beloved Mother (Late Smt. Rekha Sinha) for whom I am sure she is in a better place. I would like to thank my beloved family members my Wife (Mrs. Seema Sinha), cutiepie Daughter (Ms. Shreenika Sinha), younger brother (Mr. Yashwant Sinha) along with his wife (Mrs. Neha), and my Father (Mr. Siltu Sinha) with whose support I was able to complete my dream book.

My favorite dictum is *'Give a person a fish and they'll eat for one day; teach them how to catch their own and they'll be fed forever'*.

Disclaimer

It is my sincere endeavour to accumulate and compile information on various topics of Drugs, Medical Devices, Registered Medical Practitioner (RMPs) and Qualified Persons (like Registered Pharmacist, Competent Person and Competent Technical Staff) prescribed in the Drugs and Cosmetics Act and Rules thereunder. The subject information in this book is in convenience of readers not limited to the pharmacists, offline or online pharmacies, medical devices bussiness owners to the best of my knowledge and with my substantial experience in the field of Pharmacy since 2011.

All the information of this book is for knowledge and educational purposes only. These topics and relative text are covered to highlight the important points and topics related to the licensed products which includes Allopathic medicines, Homeopathic medicines and Medical Devices including IVDs (In-Vitro Diagnostics). The topics covered in this book are attributed to the interpretations of the law of the land related to the Drugs and Medical devices having references of correct sources, i.e., Drugs and Cosmetics Act and Rules, other books, Manuscripts, Websites, Electronic media, Review articles, Research articles, White papers, Lectures, et al.

Contents

Chapter 1: Introduction to the Drugs and Cosmetics Act, 1940 and Rules .. 1

Chapter 2: Drug Regulatory Authorities and their Powers 9

Chapter 3: Allopathic Drugs and Schedules 18

Chapter 4: Allopathic Drugs Sale Rule.. 59

Chapter 5: Homeopathic Medicines and Sale Rules 74

Chapter 6: Medical Devices and In Vitro Diagnostics (IVDs) Sale Rule 81

Chapter 7: Registered Medical Practitioner (RMP) and Medicine Prescribing... 97

Chapter 8: Registered Pharmacist (RP) and Prescription Drugs Dispensing 102

Chapter 9: Part VI - Sale of Drugs other than Homeopathic Medicines .. 112

Chapter 10: New Law Reforms related to the Drugs and Pharmacy 143

CHAPTER 1

Introduction to the Drugs and Cosmetics Act, 1940 and Rules

Evolution of the Drugs and Cosmetics Act, 1940

The Drugs and Cosmetics Act was formed before Indian independence during British rule. It was under the Act 23 of 1940 under the Government of India Act, 1935 later known as the 'Drugs Act, 1940'. Before independent India, the 'Drugs' was covered under the *'List 2 of 7th Schedule of the Government of India Act, 1935'*. All legislatures of provinces passed a resolution, wherein Central Legislature was authorized to legislate for regulating the import, manufacture, distribution and sale of drugs, that gave birth to the Drug Act, 1940.

Chopra Commission (1930-1931): In 1930, an expert committee was formed after consulting with provincial governments and its people to learn and analyze the loop-holes in the quality of Indian drugs that were being sold in India. This committee was headed by Lt. Col. R. N. Chopra (*Father of Indian Pharmacology*). The Chopra Commission submitted its report in 1931 thereby recommending enactment of India legislation for the control of Drugs and Pharmacy either as a combined Act or a separate Drugs Act and Pharmacy Act. Finally, the 'Drugs Act' received assent of the Governor General in Council, on 10th April, Act 23 of 1940.

Post Independence Era: After independence of India, the *'Article 246'* of the Constitution of India gave law making powers upon some specific subjects to the Parliament and State legislatures. The *'Seventh (7th) Schedule'* to the Constitution provides *'Central list - List I'*, *'State list - II'* and *'Concurrent list - III'*. For any subject on the *'Concurrent list'* both the Central and the State Government can legislate. Drugs are enlisted on SN. 19 of the *'Concurrent list'* as *'19. Drugs and poisons, subject to the provisions of entry 59 of List I with respect to opium'*. Hence, both the Central and the State Government has power to legislate and amend this subject. In 1962, the word 'Cosmetics' was added in the 'Drugs Act, 1940' thereafter the Act was renamed as 'Drugs and Cosmetics Act, 1940'.

Provisions under the Drugs and Cosmetics Act

All provisions under this Act are placed suitably in 5 Chapters for better understanding and enforcement by the regulators. Details under the Chapter includes:

Chapter	Parts covered
Chapter I	Short title, extend, commencement and definitions of drugs and others
Chapter II	Drugs Technical Advisory Board (DTAB) and other committees
*Chapter III	Import of the Drugs and Cosmetics
**Chapter IV	Manufacture, Sale, and Distribution of the Drugs and Cosmetics
Chapter IV-A	Provisions relating to Ayurvedic, Siddha and Unani (ASU) Drugs
Chapter V	Miscellaneous - Power to give directions, Offences and Penalities

NOTE: **Chapter IV shall take effect in a particular State only from such notification as given by the State Government and *Chapter III shall come into as date of notification by the Central Government.

Objectives of the Drugs and Cosmetics Act and Rules

- To regulate the import, manufacture, distribution and sale of drugs, medical devices and cosmetics through licensing.
- To ensure that manufacture, distribution and sale of drugs, medical devices and cosmetics is done under the supervision of the qualified persons (like registered pharmacists or competent persons).
- To prevent substandard in drugs, presumably for maintaining high standards of medical treatment.
- To regulate the manufacture and sale of Ayurvedic, Siddha, Unani (ASU) and Homeopathic (H) medicines.

- To prevent import of substandard or counterfeit drugs and prohibition of the manufacture of inferior or counterfeit drugs in the country.
- To establish Drugs Technical Advisory Board (DTAB) and Drugs Consultative Committees (DCC) for Allopathic and allied drugs, medical devices and cosmetics.
- To have drug inspectors visit licensed premises regularly.
- To control the standards of pharmaceuticals and cosmetics by collecting samples and studying them in recognised laboratories regularly.
- To make special regulations to govern the preparation, standardization, and storage of biological and special products, as well as to prescribe how various classes of medications and cosmetics should be labelled and packed.

Important Definition covered under the Drugs and Cosmetics Act

Section	About	Definition
Chapter-I Section 3(a)	Definitions of the 'Ayurvedic, Siddha, Unani Drug'	'Ayurvedic, Siddha or Unani drug' includes all medicines intended for internal or external use for or in the diagnosis, treatment, mitigation or prevention of disease or disorder in human beings or animals, and manufactured exclusively in accordance with the formulae described in, the authoritative books of Ayurvedic, Siddha and Unani Tibb systems of medicine specified in the First Schedule.
Chapter-I Section 3(aaa)	Definition of 'Cosmetic'	'Cosmetic' means any article intended to be rubbed, poured, sprinkled or sprayed on, or introduced into, or otherwise applied to, the human body or any part thereof for cleansing, beautifying, promoting attractiveness, or altering the appearance, and includes any article intended for use as a component of cosmetic.
Chapter-I	Definition of	'Drug' includes

Section 3(b)	'Drug'	(i) all medicines for internal or external use of human beings or animals and all substances intended to be used for or in the diagnosis, treatment, mitigation or prevention of any disease or disorder in human beings or animals, including preparations applied on human body for the purpose of repelling insects like mosquitoes, (ii) such substances (other than food) intended to affect the structure or any function of the human body or intended to be used for the destruction of [vermin] or insects which cause disease in human beings or animals, as may be specified from time to time by the Central Government by notification in the Official Gazette, (iii) all substances intended for use as components of a drug including empty gelatin capsules, and (iv) such devices intended for internal or external use in the diagnosis, treatment, mitigation or prevention of disease or disorder in human beings or animals, as may be specified from time to time by the Central Government by notification in the Official Gazette, after consultation with the Board.
Part-I Section 2(dd)	Definition of 'Homeopathic medicines'	Homeopathic medicines include any drug which is recorded in Homeopathic provings or therapeutic efficacy of which has been established through long clinical experience as recorded in authoritative Homeopathic literature of India and abroad and which is prepared according to the techniques of Homeopathic pharmacy and covers combination of ingredients of such Homeopathic medicines but does not include a medicine which is administered by parenteral route.
Part-I	Definition of	Registered medical practitioner means a

Section 2(ee)	'Registered Medical Practitioner (RMP)'	person: (i) Holding a qualification granted by an authority specified or notified under section 3 of the Indian Medical Degrees Act, 1916 (7 of 1916), or specified in the Schedules to the Indian Medical Council Act, 1956 (102 of 1956), or (ii) Registered or eligible for registration in a medical register of a State meant for the registration of persons practising the modern scientific system of medicine excluding the Homeopathic system of medicine, or (iii) registered in a medical register other than a register for the registration of Homeopathic practitioner of a State, who although not falling within sub-clause (i) or sub-clause (ii) is declared by a general or special order made by the State Government in this behalf as a person practicing the modern scientific system of medicine for the purposes of this Act, or (iv) registered or eligible for registration in the register of dentists for a State under the Dentists Act, 1948 (16 of 1948), or (v) who is engaged in the practice of veterinary medicine and who possesses qualifications approved by the State Government.
Part-I Section 2(f)	Definition of 'Retail Sale' in pharmacy	Sale whether to a hospital, or dispensary, or a medical, educational or research institute or to any other person other than a sale by way of wholesale dealing.
Part-I Section 2(g)	Definition of 'Wholesale' in pharmacy	Sale to a person for the purpose of selling again and includes sale to a hospital, dispensary, medical, educational or research institution.
Chapter-I Section 3(b)(iv)	Definition of 'Medical Device' under the Drugs	All devices including an instrument, apparatus, appliance, implant, material or other article, whether used alone or in

	and Cosmetics Act	combination, including a software or an accessory, intended by its manufacturer to be used specially for human beings or animals which does not achieve the primary intended action in or on human body or animals by any pharmacological or immunological or metabolic means, but which may assist in its intended function by such means for one or more of the specific purposes of: a) Diagnosis, prevention, monitoring, treatment or alleviation of any disease or disorder; or b) Diagnosis, monitoring, treatment, alleviation or assistance for, any injury or disability; or c) Investigation, replacement or modification or support of the anatomy or of a physiological process; or d) Supporting or sustaining life; or e) Disinfection of medical devices; or f) Control of conception.
Chapter-I Section 3(zb)	Definition of 'Medical Device' under the Medical Devices Rules, 2017	(A) substances used for in vitro diagnosis and surgical dressings, surgical bandages, surgical staples, surgical sutures, ligatures, blood and blood component collection bag with or without anticoagulant covered under sub clause (i), (B) substances including mechanical contraceptives (condoms, intrauterine devices, tubal rings), disinfectants and insecticides notified in the Official Gazette under sub-clause (ii), (C) devices notified from time to time under section 3(b)(iv) of the Drugs and Cosmetics Act, 1940. *Explanation: For the purpose of these rules, substances used for in vitro diagnosis shall be referred to as in vitro diagnostic medical devices* .
Chapter-I	Definition of 'In	IVDs are substances intended to be used

Section 3(zb)	vitro diagnostic - IVD kits' under the Medical Devices Rules	outside human or animal bodies for the diagnosis of any disease or disorder in human beings or animals covered under section 3(b)(i) of the Drugs and Cosmetics Act, 1940, and IVDs that are notified from time to time, as a device under section 3(b)(iv) of the Drugs and Cosmetics Act, 1940.
Section 2(i) of Pharmacy Act, 1948	Definition of 'Registered Pharmacist'	'Registered Pharmacist' means a person who is a registered Pharmacist as defined in clause (i) of section (2) of the Pharmacy Act, 1948 (Act No. 8 of 1948).
Drugs Rule 64(2)	Definition of 'Competent Person' (for sale of drugs)	(a) Is a Registered Pharmacist; or (b) Has passed the matriculation examination or its equivalent examination from a recognised Board with four years' experience in dealing with sale of drugs; or (c) Holds a degree of a recognised University with one year's experience in dealing with drugs.
Medical Devices Rule 87(A)(3)(v)	Definition of 'Competent Technical Staff' (for sale of medical devices)	(a) Hold a degree from a recognized University/Institution; or (b) Is a registered pharmacist; or (c) Has passed intermediate examination or its equivalent examination from a recognised Board with one-year experience in dealing with sale of medical devices.
Drugs Rule 67(f)	Definition of 'Competent Person' (competent to deal in Homeopathic medicines)	(a) Degree in Homoeopathy from a recognized University; or (b) Degree in pharmacy (B.Pharm) from a recognized University; or (c) Bachelor's degree (Graduate) from a recognized University with one-year experience of dealing in Homeopathic medicines in the premises of a registered Homoeopathic Medical Practitioner or premises holding license in Form 20C or Form 20D; or

| | | (d) Diploma in Homeopathic Pharmacy; or
(e) Diploma in Homeopathy Medicine and Surgery. |
| --- | --- | --- |

Difference between a 'Drug' and 'Medicine': The Drugs and Cosmetics Act and Rules thereunder, does not define or distinguish the terms 'drug' and 'medicine'. In common understanding a 'Drug' is in the form of crude, raw or pure substance as such and is often called the active ingredient. When this drug is converted into a dosage form like 'tablet' or 'syrup' it becomes a 'medicine'.

For example 'Paracetamol/Acetaminophen' is a 'Drug' and when it is made in the form of a 'tablet' or 'syrup' then it becomes a 'Medicine' making it fit for consumption. However, in the Drugs and Cosmetics Act and Rules majority of the terminology used is 'Drug' only.

CHAPTER 2

Drug Regulatory Authorities and their Powers

Powers of the Central Government

In excise of the powers conferred by Sections 12, 33 and 33(N) of the Drugs and Cosmetics Act, 1940 (23 of 1940), the Central Government has power to frame rules and make necessary amendments therein from time to time in interest of public for total quality management of drugs. Necessary schedules are also made to these Rules. Some of the Rules and amendments under this provisions are:

- The Drugs Rules, 1945
- The Medical Devices Rules, 2017
- The New Drugs and Clinical Trials Rules, 2019 and
- The Cosmetics Rules, 2020

Drug Regulatory Authorities

SN	Classification	Regulatory Bodies
1	Advisory Wing	1. <u>Drugs Technical Advisory Board (DTAB)</u> - 18 members board nominated by the Central Government who takes the policy decisions pertaining to technical aspects of the Drugs and Cosmetics Act and Rules and sends the recommendations to the Ministry of Health and Family Welfare, Government of India for its approval. 2. <u>Drugs Consultative Committee (DCC)</u> - Nominated by the Central Government for advising the Central and State Governments, as well as, the DTAB on

			the matters pertaining to the uniform implementation of the provisions of Drugs Act and Rules.
2	Analytical Wing	1.	<u>Central Drugs Laboratory (CDL)</u> - Takes, and analyse the sample of the drugs or cosmetics along with advising the Central Government and the State Governments and Union Territories on the matters pertaining to the analysis of drugs and cosmetics.
		2.	<u>State Drug Control Laboratory</u> - Analytical quality control of drug and cosmetics manufactured within the country on behalf of the Central and State Drug Controller Administrations.
		3.	<u>Government Analysts</u> - Appointed by Central Government and State Government for the purpose of test or analysis of drugs and cosmetics. They are employed in Central Drugs Laboratory and Drug Testing Laboratories of States and Union Territories.
3	Administrative Wing	1.	<u>Drug Licensing authorities</u> - The qualification required for Licensing Authority is a graduate in pharmacy or pharmaceutical chemistry or in medicine with clinical pharmacology or microbiology from a university established in India and a minimum of 5 years in manufacturing or testing of drugs or enforcement of the provisions of the Act.
		2.	<u>Drug Control authorities</u> - Regulatory Control over the manufacture, distribution and sales of drugs & cosmetics and to maintain standard of drugs, medical devices & cosmetics.
		3.	<u>Drug inspectors</u> - Appointed by the State Government and Central Government to regularly inspect the drug, medical devices or cosmetics manufacturing unit and retail/wholesale pharmacy including medical devices bussiness and manufacturing premises regularly with the responsibility of ensuring strict implementation of Drugs and Cosmetics Act in the area of his/her jurisdiction.

Role of Central and State Government as a Drug Regulator

The architecture of drug regulation in India is designed as a classic command and control system in which the regulator prescribes standards, distributes licenses and then undertakes inspection to check for compliance. Hence, both the central and the state governments are identified as regulators under the Drugs and Cosmetics Act.

Central Government Power

The Ministry of Health and Family Welfare (MOHFW) represents the central government in this regard where the Director General of Health Services (DGHS) oversees the regulatory functions of the MOHFW. Under the DGHS, the CDSCO holds the final delegation of regulatory responsibility. The CDSCO is a non-statutory body, and not independent of the MOHFW. The CDSCO has its head office at New Delhi with six zonal offices, four sub zonal offices, thirteen Port offices and seven laboratories. The CDSCO is headed by the Drugs Controller General of India (DCGI).

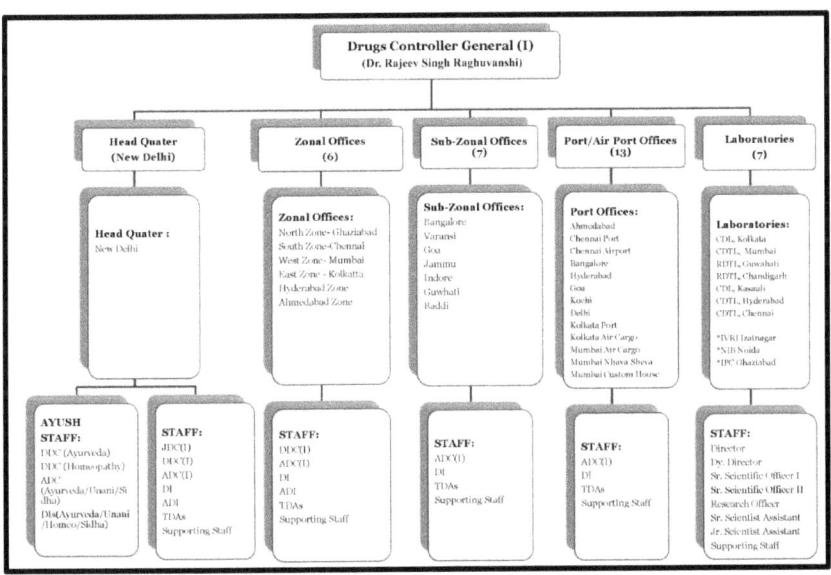

Fig: Organization Chart of CDSCO

The main functions of the Central Government related to Drugs, Cosmetics and Medical Devices includes:

- Approval of any 'New drugs' and 'New medical devices'
- Registration and control of imported drugs

- Approvals for clinical trials
- Laying down standards for drugs, cosmetics, diagnostics and medical devices
- Approval of licenses for high risk products (large volume parenterals, vaccines and biotechnology products and operation of blood banks)
- Coordinating activities of the states and advising them on matters of uniformity in regulatory administration in the implementation of the Act, and
- Grant of manufacturing license for the Class-C and Class-D medical devices.

State Government Power

Every State and Union Territory (UT) of India has its own State Food and Drug Administration (FDA) or State Drug Control Department whose duty is to ensure efficacy, safety and quality of the drugs, cosmetics and medical devices. This agency also monitors whether the price of medicines and medical devices are as per the fixed prices by the NPPA (National Pharmaceutical Pricing Authority) as per the DPCO (Drug Price Control Order, 2013). Hence, this department ensures that any retailer, wholesaler, stockist, dealer or manufacturer does not sell drugs or medical devices beyond the price fixed by the NPPA (National Pharmaceutical Pricing Authority) as per the DPCO (Drug Price Control Order) latest price fixation.

The main functions of State Government includes:

- Licensing of manufacturing establishments and sale premises of drugs and medical devices,
- Undertaking inspections of such premises to ensure compliance with license conditions,
- Drawing samples for testing and monitoring of quality of drugs,
- Taking actions like suspension/cancellation of state sale or manufacturing licenses of drugs and medical devices,
- Surveillance over sale of spurious and adulterated drugs,
- Instituting legal prosecution when required and monitoring of objectionable advertisements for drugs, and
- Grant of manufacturing license for the Class A and B medical devices.

Types of healthcare products or services controlled and regulated by the State FDA (Food and Drug Adminstartion) or State Drug Control Department includes:

- Allopathic Drugs - Sale and manufacture.
- Homeopathic Drugs - Sale and manufacture.
- Medical Devices including IVD (in vitro diagnostic) - Sale and manufacture.
- Ayurvedic, Siddha and Unani Drugs - Manufacture only.
- Cosmetics - Manufacture only.
- Blood, Blood component and Blood products - Sale only.

NOTE: *Many Indian states have a separate State AYUSH drug control department which grants manufacturing license for ayurvedic, siddha, unani, homeopathic drugs, and sale license for the homeopathic drugs.*

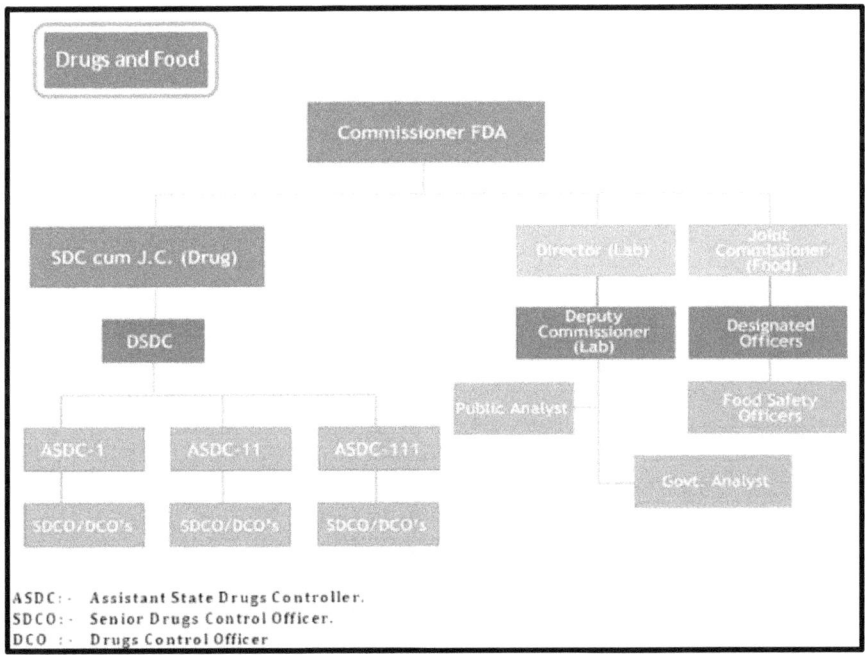

Fig 2: State FDA / Drug Control Department Organization Structure

Drug Inspector (DI)

The Drug Inspectors are appointed both by the State   Government and Central Government for specific jurisdiction areas or for specific category of activity. There could be a set of inspectors exclusively for the manufacturing of drug formulations. Drug Inspector works under the Drug Controlling Authority under State Government or Central Government as the case may be. A Drug Inspector has been charged with the responsibility of ensuring strict implementation of Drugs and Cosmetics Act in the area of his/her. jurisdiction area.

Difference between Drug Inspector (DI) and Police Inspector

The Drugs and Cosmetics Act, 1940 specifies and defines the powers of the Drug Inspector (DI) under the Section 22. It is important to note that Drug Inspectors are different from the Police Inspectors.

SN	Drug Inspector (DI)	Police Inspector
1	Appointment by the State Drug Control Department or CDSCO reporting to the Health Department (at State level) or Ministry of Health (CDSCO at Central level).	Appointed by the State Home Department.
2	Investigate in matters related to drugs, cosmetics and medical devices.	Maintain peace and stability or law order in that state.
3	Can file an FIR for the offenses committed under violation of the Chapter IV of the Drugs and Cosmetics Act.	Can register an FIR for a cognizable offense but, cannot file an FIR for the offenses committed under Chapter IV of the Drugs and Cosmetics Act.
4	Can search, investigate, raid and file complaint against the individual or firm in case of the violation of the Drugs and Cosmetics Act.	Cannot file compliant against an individual or firm in case of the violation of the Drugs and Cosmetics Act but, can assist and provide security assistance to the Drug Inspectors in case help in sought by the Drug Control Department.

Qualification for Drug Inspector (DI)

Every Drug Inspector shall be deemed to be a public servant under Section 21 of the Indian Penal Code (IPC). Following are the qualification criteria for a Drug Inspector:

- The person should not have direct or indirect financial interest in any of the activities concerned with import, manufacturing, sale or distribution of drugs.
- A 'graduate in pharmacy' or 'pharmaceutical sciences' or 'medicine' with specialization in 'clinical pharmacology' or 'microbiology' from a University established in India, is eligible for the post of Inspector.
- For the purpose of Schedules C and C (1) drugs:
  - Atleast 18 months of experience in manufacturing of atleast one substance specified in Schedules C and C (1) **or**,
  - Atleast 3 years experience in inspecting the firms manufacturing Schedules C and C (1) drugs **or**,
  - Atleast 18 months experience in testing of atleast one of the substances in schedules C and C (1) in a laboratory approved for the purpose.

NOTE: The requirement of these qualifications shall not, however, apply to those persons appointed as Inspector on or before 18th October, 1993.

Duties of Drug Inspectors at sale and manufacturing premise

Subject to instructions of the Controlling Authority, it shall be the duty of an Inspector authorised to inspect sale and manufacturing premises licensed for the sale or manufacturing of drug and cosmetics . Following are the duties of the Drug Inspector:

- Inspect any manufacturing or sale premise not less than once a year and satisfy himself that conditions of licenses are being observed.
- Search any person, premise, vehicle, vessel or other conveyance which he believes is being used for the offense or violations of the Act.
- Examine and seize any record, register, document or any other material object/s found with any person, vehicle, place, vessel or other conveyance as an evidence of an offense punishable under this Act or the rules made thereunder.

- Procure and send the seized sample like drugs or cosmetics for test or analysis if he has reason to suspect that drug is sold or stocked in contravention with provisions of the Act or Rules.
- Investigate any complaint received to him in the form of writing, mail, message or call.
- Maintain a record of inspections.
- Make necessary enquiries whenever he feels is in offense or violation of the Act.
- Institute prosecutions in respect of breaches of the Act and Rules.
- Detain the imported packages which he has reason to believe contain drugs, the import of which is prohibited.

Procedure to be followed by a Drug Inspector while collecting seized samples from a 'sale premise': The sample withdrawn or seized from drugs or cosmetics sale stores should be divided into 4 parts. The seizure of medicine should be carried out in accordance with the Code of Criminal Procedure, 1898 in presence of witnesses. The samples should be sealed and the seal of the drug store owner should also be allowed. In case of injectables, 4 different ampoules of the same batch are seized. The payment of fair price of seized material is made to the drug store owner and the receipt is prepared by Drug Inspector separately and the form is filled up. Any action of seizure or raid is required to be informed to the Judicial Magistrate of that area immediately within 24 hours.

Out of 4 samples confiscated:

- <u>First sample</u> - Inspector
- <u>Second sample</u> - Government analyst
- <u>Third sample</u> - Drugs/Cosmetics store owner
- <u>Fourth sample</u> - Manufacturer

The sample sent by an Inspector to Government Analyst shall be by registered post or by hand in sealed packet enclosed with memorandum in "**Form 18**" in an outer cover addressed to the Government Analyst. A copy of memorandum and a specimen impression of seal is sent separately to the Government Analyst by registered post.

Procedure to be followed by Drug Inspector while collecting seized samples from a 'manufacturing premise': In case of raid or seizure of medicine or cosmetics at manufacturing premise, 3 seized samples are prepared:

- <u>First sample</u> - Inspector
- <u>Second sample</u> - Manufacturer
- <u>Third sample</u> - Government Analyst

After receipt of report of analysis, action is taken accordingly. If the report is satisfactory, regular sale is allowed. If it is not satisfactory, further legal action is taken up. Any physical assault or a threat in writing or on telephone to Inspector while discharging his duties is considered as an offence punishable with imprisonment upto 3 years or fine or both.

Form No.	Description
15	Order given by Inspector requiring a person not to dispose of any stock in his possession.
16	Receipt the Inspector tenders for the seized material.
17	Intimation to the person from whom the sample is taken.
17A	Receipts of samples of drugs/cosmetics taken where fair price is tendered.
18	Memorandum to be sent by Drug Inspector to the Government analyst for the purpose of analysis of seized formulation.

Table: Important forms to be filled after seizure of the sample by the Drug Inspector.

CHAPTER 3

Allopathic Drugs and Schedules

Introduction

The Drugs Rules has provisions for classification of allopathic drugs under given schedules and there are guidelines on the basis of the following criterias of each medicines:

- Storage condition,
- Sale, stock and distribution,
- Display requirement and,
- Prescription requirement.

Drugs Rules	Description
Rule 61	Forms of licenses to sell drugs (Allopathic drugs)
Rule 62	Sale at more than one place (Allopathic drugs)
Rule 63	Duration of sale license (Allopathic drugs)
Rule 64	Conditions to be satisfied before a license in Form 20, 20B, 20F, 20G, 21 or 21B is granted or renewed (Allopathic drugs)
Rule 65	Condition of licenses (Allopathic drugs)
Rule 66	Cancellation and suspension of licenses (Allopathic drugs)
Rule 96	Manner of Labeling (manner on the label of the innermost container of

	any drug and on every other covering in which the container is packed)
Rule 97	Labeling of allopathic drugs (container of a medicine for internal use)

Table: Notable Drugs Rules for Allopathic drugs covered under the Drugs and Cosmetics Act, 1940

Allopathic Drugs Schedule

In India as per the Drugs Rules the list of Schedule has been alloted alphabetically namely:

- Schedule A: Application forms and license types.
- Schedule B: Fees for test or analysis by the Central Drugs Laboratories or State Drugs Laboratories.
- Schedule B1: Fees for the test or analysis by the pharmacopeia laboratory for Indian medicine or the government analyst.
- Schedule C: Biological and Special Products.
- Schedule C(1): Other Special Products.
- Schedule D: Import requirements.
- Schedule D(1): Information and undertaking required to be submitted by the manufacturer or his authorized agent with the Application Form for a Registration Certificate.
- Schedule D(2): Information required to be submitted by the manufacturer or his authorized agent with the Application Form for the registration of a bulk drug/formulation/special product for its import into India.
- Schedule D(3): Information and undertaking required to be submitted by the manufacturer or his authorised importer/distributor/agent with the application form for a registration certificate.
- Schedule E(1): List of poisonous substances under the Ayurvedic (including Siddha) and Unani Systems of Medicine.
- Schedule F: Part XII B describes the requirements for the functioning and operation of a blood bank and/or for preparation of blood components. Part XII D describes the requirements for collection, processing, testing, storage, banking and release of umbilical cord blood derived stem cells.

- Schedule F1: Part 1 describes vaccines. Part 2 describes the antisera. Part 3 details about Diagnostic antigens which describes the provisions applicable to the Manufacture and Standardization of Diagnostic Agents (Bacterial Origin) . Part 4 mentions General.
- Schedule F2: Standards for surgical dressings.
- Schedule F3: Standards for umbilical tapes.
- Schedule FF: Standards for ophthalmic preparations.
- Schedule G: List of drugs which are mostly hormonal in nature.
- Schedule H: List of drugs which can be sold out in retail against prescription of registered medical practitioner only i.e. prescription drugs.
- Schedule H1: List of drugs which can be sold out in retail against prescription of registered medical practitioner only. This schedule contains mostly antibiotics and habit forming drugs.
- Schedule H2: List of 300 allopathic branded drugs that falls under Schedule H2 for which QR/Bar code on drug label is mandatory including both prescription and non-prescription allopathic drugs.
- Schedule I: Omitted.
- Schedule J: List of diseases and ailments (by whatever name described) which a drug may not purport to prevent or cure or make claims to prevent or cure.
- Schedule K: Class of drugs and extent & condition of exemption from provisions of Drug and Cosmetic Act, 1940 & Rules therunder.
- Schedule L: Omitted.
- Schedule L1: Good laboratory practices and requirements of premises and equipment's.
- Schedule M: Good manufacturing practices and requirements of premises, plant and equipment for pharmaceutical products. Sub parts of Schedule M includes:
  - Part 1: Good manufacturing practices for premises and materials
  - Part 1A: Specific requirements for manufacture of sterile products, parenteral preparations (small volume injectables and large volume parenterals) and sterile ophthalmic preparations.
  - Part 1B: Specific requirements for manufacture of oral solid dosage forms (tablets and capsules)

- Part 1C: Specific requirements for manufacture of oral liquids (syrups, elixirs, emulsions and suspensions)
- Part 1D: Specific requirements for manufacture of topical products, i.e. external preparations (creams, ointments, pastes, emulsions, lotions, solutions, dusting powders and identical products)
- Part 1E: Specific requirements for manufacture of metered-dose-inhalers (mdi)
- Part 1F: Specific requirements of premises, plant and materials for manufacture of active pharmaceutical ingredients (bulk drugs)
- Part 2: Requirements of plant and equipment
- Schedule M1: Good manufacturing practices and requirements of premises, plant and equipment for homeopathic medicines.
- Schedule M2: Requirements of factory premises for manufacture of cosmetics.
- Schedule M3: Quality management system for notified medical devices and in-vitro diagnostics.
- Schedule N: List of minimum equipment for the efficient running of a 'Pharmacy' where drug is both compounded and dispensed (not applicable for 'Chemists and Druggists' where drug is only dispensed).
- Schedule O: Standard for disinfectant fluids. Sub parts of Schedule O includes:
  - Part 1: Provision applicable to black fluids and white fluids
  - Part 2: Provisions applicable to other disinfectant fluids
- Schedule P: Life period of drugs.
- Schedule P1: Pack size of drugs.
- Schedule Q: List of dye, colour and pigments
  - Part 1: List of dyes, colours and pigments permitted to be used in cosmetics and soaps
  - Part 2: List of colours permitted to be used in soaps
- Schedule R: Standards for condoms made of rubber latex intended for single use and other mechanical contraceptives.
- Schedule R1: Indian Standards laid down from time to time by the Bureau of Indian Standards for medical devices.

- Schedule S: Standards for Cosmetics Standards laid down from time to time by the Bureau of Indian Standards.
- Schedule T: Good manufacturing practices for ayurvedic, siddha and unani (ASU) medicines.
- Schedule TA: Form for record of utilization of raw material by ayurveda or siddha or unani licensed manufacturing units during the financial year.
- Schedule U: Particulars shown in manufacturing records of drugs.
- Schedule U1: Particulars shown in manufacturing record of cosmetics.
- Schedule V: Standards for patent or proprietary medicines.
- Schedule X: List of habit forming and narcotic drugs which are habit forming and likely to be misused for addictive purposes.
- Schedule Y: Requirements and guidelines for permission to import and/or manufacture of new drugs for sale or to undertake clinical trials.
- Schedule Z: Not available.

Important Schedules - Allopathic drugs

Drug Schedule	Definition	Number	Drug Label Warning (Rule 97 of Drugs Rules)
Schedule H	Drugs which can be sold on the prescription of a Allopathic Registered Medical Practitioners (RMP) only.	552	'To be sold by retail on the prescription of a Registered Medical Practioner only'.
Schedule H1	Prescription Drugs including few antibiotics, habit forming drugs, few anti TB drugs which can be abused under Schedule H with highly regulated sale.	50	- 'It is dangerous to take this preparation except in accordance with the medical advice'. - 'Not to be sold by retail without the prescription of a Registered Medical

				Practitioner'.
Schedule G	Prescription Drugs that can be administered only under supervision of a Registered Medical Practitioner (RMP).	57		*'It is dangerous to take this preparation except under medical supervision'*.
Schedule X	Prescription Drugs that are highly regulated due to its addiction and abusive nature.	16		*'To be sold by retail on the prescription of a Registered Medical Practitioner only'*.
Schedule K	Drugs that do not require a sale license or prescription for sale with certain conditions (exemption under Chapter IV of the Drugs Act). The list consists of total 39 Serial Numbers for the categories of drugs or devices including ommitted ones.	Not clearly defined		Not Applicable
Schedule J	Contains a list of diseases and ailments which an allopathic drug may not claim to prevent or cure for 51 diseases/conditions as per Drugs Rules 106.	51		Not Applicable
Schedule H2	Contains list of 300 branded allopathic prescription and non-prescription drugs in which QR/Bar code is mandatory as per the labelling requirements.	300		Not Applicable

Schedule C Allopathic Drugs (Biologicals and Special products)

Defined in Part X of the Drugs and Cosmetics Act, 1940 including Rule 23, 61 and 76 of the Drugs Rules. These are 'Biologicals and Special products' which includes following category:

1. Sera.
2. Solution of serum proteins intended for injection.
3. Vaccines for parenteral injections.
4. Toxins.
5. Antigen.
6. Antitoxins.
7. Neo-arsphenamine and analogous substances used for the specific treatment of infective diseases.
8. Insulin.
9. Pituitary (Posterior Lobe) Extract.
10. Adrenaline and Solutions of Salts of Adrenaline.
11. Antibiotics and preparations thereof in a form to be administered parenterally.
12. Any other preparation which is meant for parenteral administration as such or after being made up with a solvent or medium or any other sterile product and which requires to be stored in a refrigerator; or does not require to be stored in a refrigerator.
13. Sterilized surgical ligature and sterilized surgical suture.
14. Bacteriophages.
15. Ophthalmic preparations.
16. Sterile Disposable Devices for single use only.

Schedule C1 Allopathic Drugs (Other Special products)

Defined in Part X of the Drugs and Cosmetics Act, 1940 including Rules 23, 61 and 76 of the Drugs Rules. These are 'Other Special products' which includes following category:

1. Drugs belonging to the Digitalis group and preparations containing drugs belonging to the Digitalis group not in a form to be administered parenterally.
2. Ergot and preparations containing Ergot not in a form to be administered parenterally.
3. Adrenaline and preparations containing Adrenaline not in a form to be administered parenterally.
4. Fish Liver Oil and preparations containing Fish Liver Oil.

5. Vitamins and preparations containing any vitamins not in a form to be administered parenterally.
6. Liver extract and preparations containing liver extract not in a form to be administered parenterally.
7. Hormones and preparations containing hormones not in a form to be administered parenterally.
8. Vaccine not in a form to be administered parenterally.
9. Antibiotics and preparations thereof not in a form to be administered parenterally.
10. In-vitro Blood Grouping Sera.
11. In-vitro Diagnostic Devices for HIV, HbsAg and HCV.

Schedule G Allopathic Drugs

These are allopathic prescription drugs mostly under category of the hormonal preparations. The drug label must display the text *"Schedule G Prescription Drug - Caution: It is dangerous to take this preparation except under medical supervision"* prominently. These drug categories has to be dispensed by a retail only under the supervision of an endorsed Registered Pharmacist only.

```
Metformin Hydrochloride Tablets IP  500mg

Each uncoated tablet contains:
Metformin Hydrochloride IP         500mg

Dosage: As prescribed by the Physician.
Keep out of reach of children
```

```
SCHEDULE G PRESCRIPTION
DRUG - CAUTION
It is dangerous to take this
preparation except under
medical supervision"
```

Fig: Schedule G Drugs - Prescription Label Warning

Following drugs are classified under the Schedule G:

1. Aminopterin
2. Bleomycin
3. Busulphan; its salts
4. Carbutamide
5. Chlorambucil; its salts
6. Chlorothiazide and other derivatives of 1, 2, 4 benzothiadrazine
7. Chlorpropamide; its salts
8. Chlorthalidone and other derivatives of Chlorbenzene compound
9. Cis-Platin
10. Cyclophosphamide; its salts

11. Cytarabine
12. Daunorubicin
13. Di-Isopropyl Fluorophosphate
14. Disodium Stilboestrol Diphosphate
15. Doxorubicin Hydrochloride
16. Ethacrynic Acid; its salts
17. Ethosuximide
18. Glibenclamide
19. Hydantoin; its salts, itss derivatives, their salts
20. Insulin, all types
21. Hydroxyurea
22. Lomustine Hydrochloride
23. Mammomustine; its salts
24. Mercaptopurine; its salts
25. Metformin; its salts
26. Methsuximide
27. Mustine; its salts
28. Paramethadione
29. Phenacemide
30. Phenformin; its salts
31. 5-Phenylhydantoin, its alkyl and aryl derivatives; its salts
32. Primadone
33. Procarpazine Hydrochloride
34. Quinthazone
35. Sarcolysine
36. Sodium 2 Mercaptoethanesulfonate Tamoxifen Citrate
37. Testolactone
38. Thiotepa
39. Tolbutamide
40. Tretamine; its salts
41. Troxidone
42. Antihistaminic substances the following, their salt, their derivatives salt of their derivatives
43. Antazoline
44. Bromodiphenhydramine
45. Buclizine
46. Chlorcyclizine
47. Chlorpheniramine
48. Clemizole
49. Cyproheptadine

50. Diphenhydramine
51. Diphenyl pyraline
52. Doxylamine Succinate
53. Isothipendyl
54. Mebhydrolin Napadisylate
55. Meclozine
56. Phenindomine
57. Pheniramine
58. Promethazine
59. Thenalidine
60. Triprolidone
61. Substances being tetra-N-substituted derivatives of Ethylene Diamine or Prophylenediamine

3.4. Schedule H Allopathic Drugs: These are allopathic prescription drugs and as per the Drugs Rules 65 and 97 these drug label must display the text *"Schedule H Prescription Drug Warning: Not to be sold by retail without the prescription of a registered Medical Practitioner"* prominently. These drug categories has to be dispensed by a retail only under the supervision of an endorsed Registered Pharmacist only.

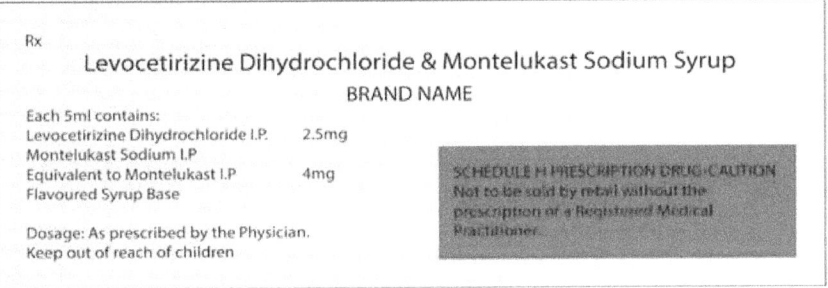

Fig: Schedule H Drugs - Prescription Label warning

For those allopathic drug which do not comes under the category of Schedule H like certain narcotic analgesics, hypnotics, sedatives, tranquillisers, corticosteroids, hormones, hypoglycemic, antimicrobials, antiepileptics, antidepressants, anticoagulants, anti-cancer drugs etc. if manufactured then, the label shall be printed with the warning or caution as the case may be for that drug covered under Schedule H.

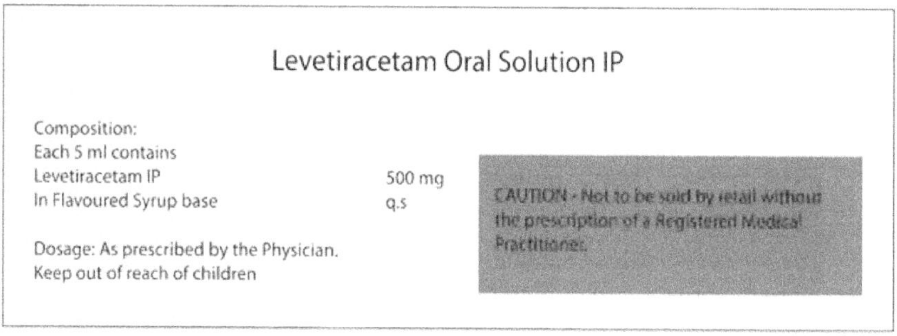

```
Levetiracetam Oral Solution IP

Composition:
Each 5 ml contains
Levetiracetam IP                          500 mg
In Flavoured Syrup base                   q.s

                                          CAUTION - Not to be sold by retail without
                                          the prescription of a Registered Medical
                                          Practitioner.

Dosage: As prescribed by the Physician.
Keep out of reach of children
```

Fig: Prescription Allopathic Drugs (not cover under Schedule H) - Prescription label warning

For those Schedule H allopathic drug which come under the preview of Narcotic Drugs and Psychotropic Substances (NDPS) Act, 1985 shall be labeled with symbol '**NRx**' in Red Colour displayed on the left top corner.

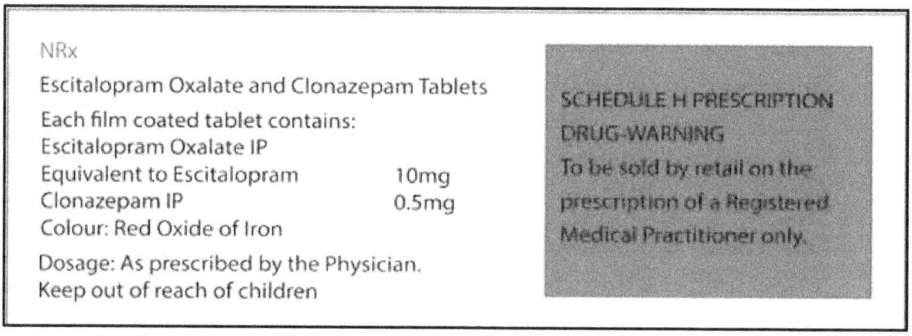

```
NRx
Escitalopram Oxalate and Clonazepam Tablets     SCHEDULE H PRESCRIPTION
Each film coated tablet contains:               DRUG-WARNING
Escitalopram Oxalate IP                         To be sold by retail on the
Equivalent to Escitalopram        10mg          prescription of a Registered
Clonazepam IP                     0.5mg         Medical Practitioner only.
Colour: Red Oxide of Iron

Dosage: As prescribed by the Physician.
Keep out of reach of children
```

Fig: Schedule H drugs (covered under the Narcotics and Psychotrophic substances - NDPS) - Prescription label warning

Till date (2023) there are 552 Schedule H Drugs namely:
1. ABACAVIR
2. ABCIXIMAB
3. ACAMPROSATE CALCIUM
4. ACEBUTOL HYDROCHLORIDE
5. ACLARUBICIN
6. ALBENDAZOLE
7. ALCLOMETASONE DIPROPIONATE
8. ACTILYSE
9. ACYCLOVIR
10. ADENOSINE
11. ADRENOCORTICOTROPHIC HORMONE (ACTH)
12. ALENDRONATE SODIUM

13. ALLOPURINOL
14. ALPHACHYMOTRYPSIN
15. ALPRAZOLAM
16. ALPROSTADIL
17. AMANTADINE HYDROCHLORIDE
18. AMIFOSTINE
19. AMIKACIN SULPHATE
20. AMILORIDE HYDROCHLORIDE
21. AMINEPTINE
22. AMINOGLUTETHIMIDE
23. AMINOSALICYLIC ACID
24. AMIODARONE HYDROCHLORIDE
25. AMITRIPTYLINE
26. AMLODIPINE BESYLATE
27. AMOSCANATE
28. AMOXOPINE
29. AMRINONE LACTATE
30. ANALGIN
31. ANDROGENIC ANABOLIC, OESTROGENIC & PROGESTATIONAL SUBSTANCES
32. ANTIBIOTICS
33. APRACLONIDINE
34. APROTININ
35. ORGANIC COMPOUND OF ARSENIC
36. ARTEETHER
37. ARTEMETHER
38. ARTESUNATE
39. ARTICAINE HYDROCHLORIDE
40. ATENOLOL
41. ATRACURIUM BESYLATE INJECTION
42. ATORVASTATIN
43. AURANOFIN
44. AZATHIOPRINE
45. AZTREONAM
46. BACAMPICILLIN
47. BACLOFEN
48. BALSALAZIDE
49. BAMBUTEROL
50. BARBITURIC ACID
51. BASILIXIMAB

52. BENAZEPRIL HYDROCHLORIDE
53. BENIDIPINE HYDROCHLORIDE
54. BENSERAZIDE HYDROCHLORIDE
55. BETAHISTINE DIHYDROCHLORIDE
56. BETHANIDINE SULPHATE
57. BEZAFIBRATE
58. BICALUTAMIDE
59. BICLOTYMOL
60. BIFONAZOLE
61. BIMATOPROST
62. BIPERIDEN HYDROCHLORIDE
63. BIPHENYL ACETIC ACID
64. BITOSCANATE
65. BLEOMYCIN
66. PRIMONIDINE TARTRATE
67. BROMHEXINE HYDROCLORIDE
68. BROMOCRIPTINE MESYLATE
69. BUDESONIDE
70. BULAQUINE
71. BUPIVA CAINE HYDROCHLORIDE
72. BUPROPION
73. BUSPIRONE
74. BUTENAFINE HYDROCHLORIDE
75. BUTORPHANOL TARTRATE
76. CABERGOLINE
77. CALCIUM DOBESILATE
78. CANDESARTAN
79. CAPECITABINE
80. CAPTOPRIL
81. CARBIDOPA
82. CARBOCISTEINE
83. CARBOPLATIN
84. CARBOQUONE
85. CARISOPRODOL
86. L-CARNITINE
87. CARTEOLOL HYDROCHLORIDE
88. CARVEDILOL
89. CEFADROXYL
90. CEFATOXIME SODIUM
91. CEFAZOLIN SODIUM

92. CEFDINIR
93. CEFEPIME HYDROCHLORIDE
94. CEFETAMET PIVOXIL
95. CEFPIROME
96. CEFPODOXIME POX
97. CEFTAZIDIME PENTAHYDRATE
98. CEFTIZOXIME SODIUM
99. CEFUROXIME
100. CELECOXIB
101. CENTCHROMAN
102. CENTBUTINDOLE
103. CENTPROPAZINE
104. CETIRIZINE HYDROCHLORIDE
105. CHLORDIAZEPOXIDE
106. CHLORMEZANONE
107. Omitted vide GSR 790 (E) dtd 29.10.2009
108. CHLORPROMAZINE
109. CHLORZOXAZONE
110. CICLOPIROX OLAMINE
111. CIMETIDINE
112. CINNARIZINE
113. CIPROFLOXACIN HYDROCHLORIDE MONOHYDRATE / LACTATE
114. CISPLATIN
115. CITALOPRAM HYDROBROMIDE
116. CLARITHROMYCIN
117. CLAVULANIC ACID
118. CLIDINIUM BROMIDE
119. CLINDAMYCIN
120. CLOBAZAM
121. CLOBETASOL PROPENATE
122. CLOBETASONE 17-BUTYRATE
123. CLOFAZIMINE
124. CLOFIBRATE
125. CLONAZEPAM
126. CLONIDINE HYDROCHLORIDE
127. CLOPAMIDE
128. CLOPIDOGREL BISULPHATE
129. CLOSTEBOL ACETATE
130. CLOTRIMAZOLE
131. CLOZAPINE

132. CODEINE
133. COLCHICINE
134. CORTICOSTEROIDS
135. COTRIMOXAZOLE
136. CYCLANDELATE
137. CYCLOSPORINS
138. DACLIZUMAB
139. DANAZOLE
140. DAPSONE
141. DESLORATADINE
142. DESOGESTROL
143. DEXRAZOXANE
144. DEXTRANOMER
145. Omitted vide GSR 790 (E) dtd 29.10.2009
146. DEXTROPROPOXYPHENE
147. DIAZAPAM
148. DIAZOXIDE
149. DICLOFENAC SODIUM/POTASSIUM/ACID
150. DICYCLOMIN HYDROCHLORIDE
151. DIDANOSINE
152. DIGOXINE
153. DILAZEP HYDROCHLORIDE
154. DILTIAZEM
155. DINOPROSTONE
156. DIPHENOXYLATE, ITS SALTS
157. DIPIVEFRIN HYDROCHLORIDE
158. DI-SODIUM PAMIDRONATE
159. DISOPYRAMIDE
160. DOCETAXEL
161. DOMPERIDONE
162. DONEPEZIL HYDROCHLORIDE
163. DOPAMINE HYDROCHLORIDE
164. DOTHIEPIN HYDROCHLORIDE
165. DOXAPRAM HYDROCHLORIDE
166. DOXAZOSIN MESYLATE
167. DOXEPIN HYDROCHLORIDE
168. DOXORUBICIN HYDROCHLORIDE
169. DROTRECOGIN-ALPHA
170. EBASTINE
171. ECONOZOLE

172. EFAVIRENZ
173. ENALAPRIL MELEATE
174. ENFENAMIC ACID
175. EPINEPHRINE
176. EPIRUBICINE
177. EPTIFIBATIDE
178. ERGOT, ALKALOIDS OF WHETHER HYDROGENATED OR NOT, THEIR HOMOLOGOUES, SALTS
179. ESOMEPRAZOLE
180. ESTRADIOL SUCCINATE
181. ESTRAMUSTINE PHOSPHATE
182. ETANERCEPT
183. ETHACRIDINE LACTATE
184. ETHAMBUTOL HYDROCHLORIDE
185. ETHAMSYLATE
186. ETHINYLOESTRADIOL
187. ETHIONAMIDE
188. ETIDRONATE DISODIUM
189. ETODOLAC
190. ETOMIDATE
191. ETOPOSIDE
192. EXEMESTANE
193. FAMCICLOVIR
194. FAMOTIDINE
195. FENBENDAZOLE
196. FENOFIBRATE
197. FEXOFENADINE
198. FINASTERIDE
199. FLAVOXATE HYDROCHLORIDE
200. 5-FLUOROURACIL
201. FLUDARABINE
202. FLUFENAMIC ACIDS
203. FLUNARIZINE HDROCHLORIDE
204. FLUOXETINE HYDROCHLORIDE
205. FLUPENTHIXOL
206. FLUPHENAZINE ENANTHATE AND DECANOATE
207. FLURAZEPAM
208. FLURBIPROFEN
209. FLUTAMIDE
210. FLUTICASONE PROPIONATE

211. FLUVOXAMINE MALEATE
212. FORMESTANE
213. FOSFESTRIL SODIUM
214. FOSINOPRIL SODIUM
215. FOSSPHENYTOIN SODIUM
216. FOTEMUSTINE
217. GABAPENTIN
218. GALANTHAMINE HYDROBROMIDE
219. GALLAMINE, ITS SALTS, ITS QUATERNARY COMPOUND
220. GANCYCLOVIR
221. GANIRELIX
222. GATIFLOXACIN
223. GEMCITABINE
224. GEMFIBROZIL
225. GEMTUZUMAB
226. GENODEOXYCHOLIC ACID
227. GLICLAZIDE
228. GLIMEPIRIDE
229. GLUCAGON
230. GLYCOPYRROLATE
231. GLYDIAZINAMIDE
232. GOSERELIN ACETATE
233. GRANISETRON
234. GUANETHIDINE
235. GUGULIPID
236. HALOGENATED HYDROXYQUINOLINES
237. HALOPERIDOL
238. HEPARIN
239. HEPATITIS B. VACCINE
240. HYALURONIDASE
241. HYDROCORISONE 17-BUTYRATE
242. HYDROTALCITE
243. HYDROXIZINE
244. IBUPROFEN
245. IDEBENONE
246. IINDAPAMIDE
247. IMIPRAMINE
248. INDINAVIR SULPHATE
249. INDOMETHACIN
250. INSULIN HUMAN

251. INTERFERON
252. INTRAVENOUS FAT EMULSION
253. IOBITRIDOL
254. IOHEXOL
255. IOPAMIDOL
256. IOMEPROL
257. IOPROMIDE
258. IRBESARTAN
259. IRINOTECAN HYDROCHLORIDE
260. IRON PREPARATION FOR PARENTERAL USE
261. ISEPAMICINE
262. ISOCARBOXSIDE
263. ISOFLURANE
264. ISONICOTNIC ACID HYDRAZINE AND OTHER-HYDRAGINE DERIVATIVES OF ISONICOTINIC ACID
265. ISOSORBIDE DINITRATE/ MONONITRATE
266. ISOTRETINOIN
267. ISOXSUPRINE
268. ITOPRIDE
269. KETAMINE HYDROCHLORIDE
270. KETOCONAZOLE
271. KETOPROFEN
272. KETOROLAC TROMETHAMINE
273. LABETALOL HYDROCHLORIDE
274. LACIDIPINE
275. LAMIVUDINE
276. LAMOTRIGINE
277. LATANOPROST
278. LEFUNOMIDE
279. LERCANIDIPINE HYDROCHLORIDE
280. LETROZOLE
281. LEUPROLIDE ACETATE
282. LEVAMESOLE
283. LEVARTERENOL
284. LEVOBUNOLOL
285. LEVOCETIRIZINE
286. LEVODOPA
287. LEVOFLOXACIN
288. LEVOVIST
289. LIDOFLAZINE

290. LINEZPLID
291. LITHIUM CARBONATE
292. LOFEPRAMINE DECANOATE
293. LOPERAMIDE
294. LORAZEPAM
295. LOSARTAN POTASSIUM
296. LOTEPREDNOL
297. LOVASTATIN
298. LOXAPINE
299. MEBENDAZOLE
300. MEBEVERINE HYDROCHLORIDE
301. MEDROXY PROGESTERONE ACETATE
302. MEFENAMIC ACID
303. MEFLOQUINE HYDROCHLORIDE
304. MEGESTROL ACETATE
305. MEGLUMINE IOCARMATE
306. MELAGENINA
307. MELITRACEN HYDROCHLORIDE
308. MELOXICAM
309. MEPHENESIN, ITS ESTERS
310. MEPHENTERMINE
311. MEROPENAM
312. MESTEROLONE
313. METAXALONE
314. METHICILLIN SODIUM
315. METHOCARBAMOL
316. METHOTRAXATE
317. METOCLOPRAMIDE
318. METOPROLOL TARTRATE
319. METRIZAMIDE
320. METRONIDAZOLE
321. MEXILETINE HYDROCHLORIDE
322. MIANSERIN HYDROCHLORIDE
323. MICONAZOLE
324. MIDAZOLAM
325. MIFEPRISTONE
326. MILRINONE LACTATE
327. MILTEFOSINE
328. MINOCYCLINE
329. MINOXIDIL

330. MIRTAZAPINE
331. MISOPROSTOL
332. MITOXANTRONE HYDROCHLORIDE
333. MIZOLASTINE
334. MOCLOBEMIDE
335. MOMETASONE FUROATE
336. MONTELUKAST SODIUM
337. MORPHAZINAMIDE HYDROCHLORIDE
338. MOSAPRIDE
339. MOXIFLOXACIN
340. MYCOPHENOLATE MOFETIL
341. NADIFLOXACIN
342. NADOLOL
343. NAFARELIN ACETATE
344. NALIDIXIC ACID
345. NAPROXEN
346. NARCOTICS DRUGS LISTED IN NARCOTIC DRUGS & PSYCHOTROPIC SUBSTANCES ACT, 1985
347. NATAMYCIN
348. NATEGLINIDE
349. N-BUTYL-2-CYANOACRYLATE
350. NEBIVOLOL
351. NEBUMETONE
352. NELFINAVIR MESILATE
353. NETILMICIN SULPHATE
354. NEVIRAPINE
355. NICERGOLINE
356. NICORANDIL
357. NIFEDIPINE
358. NIMESULIDE
359. NIMUSTINE HYDROCHLORIDE
360. NITRAZEPAM
361. NITROGLYCERIN
362. NORETH ISTERONE ENANTHATE
363. NORFLOXACIN
364. OCTYLONIUM BROMIDE
365. OFLOXACIN
366. OLANZAPINE
367. OMEPRAZOLE
368. ORNIDAZOLE

369. ORPHENADRINE
370. ORTHOCLONE STERILE
371. OXAZEPAM
372. OXAZOLIDINE
373. OXCARBAZEPINE
374. OXETHAZAINE HYDROCHLORIDE
375. OXICONAZOLE
376. OXOLINIC ACID
377. OXPRENOLOL HYDROCHLORIDE
378. OXYBUTYNIN CHLORIDE
379. OXYFEDRINE
380. OXYMETAZOLINE
381. OXYPHENBUTAZONE
382. OXYTOCIN
383. OZOTHINE
384. PACLITAXEL
385. PANCURONIUM BROMIDE
386. PANTOPRAZOLE
387. PARA-AMINO BENZENE SULPHONAMIDE, ITS SALTS & DERIVATIVES
388. PARP-AMINO SALICYLIC ACID, ITS SALTS, ITS DERIVATIVES
389. PARECOXIB
390. PAROXETINE HYDROCHLORIDE
391. D-PENICILLAMINE
392. PENTAZOCINE
393. PENTOXIFYLLINE
394. PEPLEOMYCIN
395. PHENELZINEH SULPHATE
396. PHENOBARBITAL
397. PHENOTHIAZINE, DERIVATIVES OF AND SALTS OF ITS DERIVATIVES
398. PHENYLBUTAZINE
399. PIMOZIDE
400. PINDOLOL
401. PIOGLITAZONE HYDROCHLORIDE
402. PIRACETAM
403. PIROXICAM
404. PITUITORY GLAND, ACTIVE PRINCIPLES OF, NOT OTHERWISE SPECIFIED IN THIS SCHEDULE AND THEIR SALTS
405. POLIDOCANOL

406. POLYESTRADIOL PHOSPHATE
407. PORACTANT ALFA
408. PRAZIQUANTEL
409. PREDNIMUSTINE
410. PREDNISOLONE STEAROYLGLYCOLATE
411. PRENOXDIAZIN HYDROCHLORIDE
412. PROMAZINE HYDROCHLORIDE
413. PROMEGESTONE
414. PROPAFENONE HYDROCHLORIDE
415. PROPANOLOL HYDROCHLORIDE
416. PROPOFOL
417. PROTRISTYLINE HYDROCHLORIDE
418. PYRAZINAMIDE
419. PYRVINIUM
420. QUETIAPINE FUMERATE
421. QUINAPRIL
422. QUINIDINE SULPHATE
423. RABEPRAZOLE
424. RACECADOTRIL
425. RALOXIFENE HYDROCHLORIDE
426. RAMIPRIL HYDROCHLORIDE
427. RANITIDINE
428. RAUWOLFIA, ALKALOIDS OF, THEIR SALTS, DERIVATIVES OF THE ALKALOIDS OR RAUWOLFIA
429. REBOXETINE
430. REPAGLINIDE
431. REPROTEROL HYDROCHLORIDE
432. RILMENIDINE
433. RILUZONE
434. RISPERIDONE
435. RITONAVIR
436. RITODRINE HYDROCHLORIDE
437. RITUXIMAB
438. RIVASTIGMINE
439. ROCURONIUM BROMIDE
440. ROPINIROLE
441. ROSOXACIN
442. ROSIGLITAZONE MELEATE
443. SALBUTAMOL SULPHATE
444. SALICYL-AZO-SULPHAPYRIDINE

445. SALMON CALCITONIN
446. SAQUINAVIR
447. SATRANIDAZOLE
448. SECNIDAZOLE
449. SEPTOPAL BEADS & CHAINS
450. SERRATIOPEPTIDASE
451. SERTRALINE HYDROCHLORIDE
452. SIBUTRAMINE HYDROCHLORIDE
453. SILDENAFIL CITRATE
454. SIMVASTATIN
455. SIROLIMUS
456. SISOMICIN SULPHATE
457. S-NEOMINOPHAGEN
458. SODIUM PICOSULPHATE
459. SODIUM CROMOGLYCATE
460. SODIUM HYALURONATE
461. SODIUM VALPROATE
462. SODIUM AND MAGLUMINE IOTHALAMATES
463. SOMATOSTATIN
464. SOMATOTROPIN
465. SOTALOL
466. SPARFLOXACIN
467. SPECTINOMYCIN HYDROCHLORIDE
468. SPIRONOLACTONE
469. STAVUDINE
470. SUCRALFATE
471. SULPHADOXINE
472. SULPHAMETHOXINE
473. SULPHAMETHOXYPYRIDAZINE
474. SULPHAPHENAZOLE
475. SULPIRIDE
476. SULPROSTONE HYDROCHLORIDE
477. SUMATRIPTAN
478. TACRINE HYDROCHLORIDE
479. TAMSULOSIN HYDROCHLORIDE
480. TRAPIDIL
481. TEGASEROD MALEATE
482. TEICOPLANIN
483. TELMISARTAN
484. TEMOZOLAMIDE

485. TERAZOSIN
486. TERBUTALINE SULPHATE
487. TERFENADINE
488. TERIZIDONE
489. TERLIPRESSIN
490. TESTOSTERONE UNDECOANOATE
491. TERATOLOL HYDROCHLORIDE
492. THALIDOMIDE
493. THIACETAZONE
494. THIOCOLCHICOSIDE
495. THIOPROPAZATE, ITS SALTS
496. THYMOGENE
497. THYMOSIN-ALPHA 1
498. TIAPROFENIC ACID
499. TIBOLONE
500. TIMOLOL MALEATE
501. TINIDAZOLE
502. TIZANIDINE
503. TOBRAMYCIN
504. TOLFENAMIC ACID
505. TOPIRAMATE
506. TOPOTECAN HYDROCHLORIDE
507. TRAMADOL HYDROCHLORIDE
508. TRANEXAMIC ACID
509. TRANYLCYPROMINE, ITS SALTS
510. TRAZODONE
511. TRETINOIN
512. TRIFLUOPERAZINE
513. TRIFLUPERIDOL HYDROCHLORIDE
514. TRIFLUSAL
515. TRIMETAZIDINE DIHYDROCHLORIDE
516. TRIMIPRAMINE
517. TRIPOTASSIUM DICITRATE BISMUTHATE
518. TROMANTADINE HYDROCHLORIDE
519. UROKINASE
520. VALSARTAN
521. VASOPRESSIN
522. VECURONIUM BROMIDE
523. VENLAFAXINE HYDROCHLORIDE
524. VERAPAMIL HYDROCHLORIDE

525. VERTEPORFIN
526. VINCRISTINE SULPHATE
527. VINBLASTINE SULPHATE
528. VINDESINE SULPHATE
529. VINORELBINE TARTRATE
530. XIPAMIDE
531. ZIDOVUDINE HYDROCHLORIDE
532. ZIPRASIDONE HYDROCHLORIDE
533. ZOLEDRONIC ACID
534. ZOLPIDEM
535. ZOPICLONE
536. ZUCLOPENTHIXOL
537. ETIZOLAM
538. ALCLOMETASONE
539. BECLOMETHASONE
540. BETAMETHASONE
541. DESONIDE
542. DESOXIMETASONE
543. DEXAMETHASONE
544. DIFLORASONE DIACETATE
545. FLUOCINONIDE
546. FLUOCINOLONE ACETONIDE
547. HALOBETASOL PROPIONATE
548. HALOMETASONE
549. METHYLPREDNISONE
550. PREDNICARBATE
551. TRIAMCINOLONE ACETONIDE
552. ACITRETIN

Schedule H1 Allopathic Drugs: Schedule H1 has been introduced through gazette notification GSR 588 (E) dated 30-08-2013 containing certain third and fourth-generation antibiotics, certain habit-forming drugs and anti-TB drugs. These are prescription drugs and as per the Drugs Rules 65 and 97 these drug label must display two text label warnings - *'It is dangerous to take this preparation except in accordance with the medical advice'* and *'Not to be sold by retail without the prescription of a Registered Medical Practitioner'* prominently. These drug categories has to be dispensed by a retail only under the supervision of an endorsed Registered Pharmacist only.

```
Rx
Cefixime Tablets IP                          200 mg
Each film coated tablet contains:
Cefixime                                     IP
(as Trihydrate)
Equivalent to Anhydrous Cefixime   200 mg
Colour: Titanium Dioxide
Dosage: As prescribed by the Physician.
Keep out of reach of children

SCHEDULE H1 PRESCRIPTION
DRUG-CAUTION
-It is dangerous to take this
preparation except in
accordance with the medical
advice- Not to be sold by
retail without the prescription
of a Registered Medical
Practitioner.
```

Fig: Schedule H1 Drugs - Prescription label warning

Those Schedule H1 drugs which come under the category of the Narcotic Drugs and Psychotropic Substances (NDPS) Act, 1985 shall be labeled with symbol '**NRx**' in Red Colour and displayed prominently.

```
NRx
Alprazolam Tablets IP                        0.25 mg

Each uncoated tablet contains:
Alprazolam IP                                0.25mg
Excipients                                   q.s.

Dosage: As prescribed by the Physician.
Keep out of reach of children

SCHEDULE H1 PRESCRIPTION
DRUG-CAUTION
-It is dangerous to take this
preparation except in
accordance with the medical
advice- Not to be sold by
retail without the prescription
of a Registered Medical
Practitioner.
```

Fig: Schedule H1 Drugs (covered under Narcotic Drugs and Psychotropic Substances) - Prescription label warning

Till date (2023) there are 50 Schedule H1 Drugs namely:

1. Alprazolam
2. Balofloxacin
3. Buprenorphine
4. Capreomycin
5. Cefdinir
6. Cefditoren
7. Cefepime
8. Cefetamet
9. Cefixime
10. Cefoperazone
11. Cefotaxime

12. Cefpirome
13. Cefpodoxime
14. Ceftazidime
15. Ceftibuten
16. Ceftizoxime
17. Ceftriaxone
18. Chlorodiazepoxide
19. Clofazimine
20. Codeine
21. Cycloserine
22. Diazepam
23. Diphenoxylate
24. Doripenam
25. Ertapenem
26. Ethambutol Hydrochloride
27. Ethionamide
28. Feropenam
29. Gemifloxacin
30. Imipenem
31. Isoniazide
32. Levofloxacin
33. Meropenem
34. Midazolam
35. Moxifloxacin
36. Nitrazepam
37. Pentazocine
38. Prulifloxacin
39. Pyrazinamide
40. Rifabutin
41. Rifampicin
42. Sodium Para-aminosalicylate
43. Sparfloxacin
44. Thiacetazone
45. Tramadol
46. Zolpidem
47. Oxytocin
48. Tapentadol
49. Oseltamivir
50. Zanamivir

Schedule X Allopathic Drugs: Schedule X are allopathic drugs which are habit forming and narcotics in its nature. These categories of drugs are not considered safe for patients if taken without supervision of registered medical practitioner (RMP) and additionally these drugs can cause addiction toward these drugs if consumed for long time. If it contains a substance specified in Schedule X, it shall be labelled with the symbol '**XRx**' which shall be in red conspicuously displayed on the left top corner of the label and be also labelled with text *'Schedule X drug -Warning: To be sold by retail on the prescription of a Registered Medical Practitioner only'* under a red rectangular box.

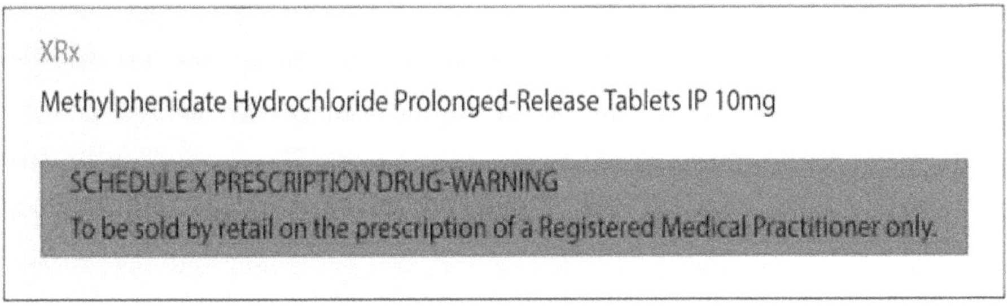

```
XRx
Methylphenidate Hydrochloride Prolonged-Release Tablets IP 10mg

SCHEDULE X PRESCRIPTION DRUG-WARNING
To be sold by retail on the prescription of a Registered Medical Practitioner only.
```

Fig: Schedule X Drug - Prescription Label Warning

Till date (2023) there are 16 Schedule X drugs namely:

1. Amobarbital
2. Amphetamine
3. Barbital
4. Cyclobarbital
5. Dexamphetamine
6. Ethchlorvynol
7. Glutethimide
8. Ketamine
9. Meprobamate
10. Methamphetamine
11. Methylphenidate
12. Methylphenobarbital
13. Pentobarbital
14. Phencyclidine
15. Phenmetrazine
16. Secobarbital

Schedule H2 Allopathic Drugs: Schedule H2 drugs are allopathic branded drugs which comprises of both prescription and non-prescription

(OTC) drugs. The list includes the top 300 brands of allopathic drugs being marketed in India. Drugs Rule 96(5)(A) mandates the manufacturers of Schedule H2 drugs to print or affix Bar code or QR code on their label. However, a retailer or wholesaler should not sale any Schedule H2 drugs which do not have QR/Bar code on its label with certain details. Following are the list of Schedule H2 drugs as on updated till 2023:

1. ACILOC 150 MG TABLET 30
2. ACILOC 300 MG TABLET 20
3. ACTEMRA 400 MG INJECTION 1
4. ACTRAPID HUMAN 40 IU INJECTION 10 ML
5. AEROCORT WITH DOSE COUNTER 50/50 MCG INHALER 200 MDI
6. AJADUO 25/5 MG TABLET 10
7. ALLEGRA 120 MG TABLET 10
8. ALLEGRA 180 MG TABLET 10
9. AMBISOME 50 MG INJECTION 20 ML
10. AMICIN 500 MG INJECTION 2 ML
11. AMLOKIND-AT 50/5 MG TABLET 10
12. ASCORIL D PLUS NEW 5/2/10 MG SYRUP 100 ML
13. ASCORIL LS 1/30/50 MG SYRUP 100 ML
14. ASCORIL PLUS 50/1.25/2 MG EXPECTORANT 120 ML
15. ASTHAKIND DX 5/2/15 MG SYRUP 100 ML
16. ASTHALIN 100 MCG INHALER 200 MDI
17. AUGMENTIN DUO 500/125 MG TABLET 10
18. AVOMINE 25 MG TABLET 10
19. AXCER 90 MG TABLET 14
20. AZEE 500 MG TABLET 5
21. AZITHRAL 500 MG TABLET 5
22. BECOSULES CAPSULE 20
23. BECOSULES Z CAPSULE 20
24. BETADINE 10 % OINTMENT 20 GM
25. BETADINE 10 % SOLUTION 100 ML
26. BETADINE MINT 2 % GARGLE 100 ML
27. BETNESOL 0.5 MG TABLET 20
28. BETNOVATE C 0.1/3 % CREAM 30 GM
29. BETNOVATE N 0.1/0.5 % CREAM 20 GM
30. BETNOVATE N 0.1/0.5 % CREAM 25 GM
31. BETT 0.5 ML INJECTION 0.5 ML
32. BEVON SYRUP 200 ML
33. BIO D3 MAX 500 MG/0.25MCG/400MCG/120MG CAPSULE 15

34. BRILINTA 90 MG TABLET 14
35. BRO ZEDEX 50/1.25/4 MG SYRUP 100 ML
36. BUDECORT 0.5 MG RESPULES 2 ML
37. CALCIROL 60000 IU GRANULES 1 GM
38. CALDIKIND PLUS 500 MG/0.25MCG/400MCG/60MG CAPSULE 10
39. CALPOL 500 MG TABLET 15
40. CALPOL 650 MG TABLET 15
41. CALPOL PEAD 250 MG SUSPENSION 60 ML
42. CANDIFORCE 200 MG CAPSULE 7
43. CCM 250 MG TABLET 40
44. CEFAKIND 500 MG TABLET 10
45. CEFTUM 500 MG TABLET 4
46. CEPODEM 200 MG TABLET 10
47. CHYMORAL FORTE 100000 IU TABLET 20
48. CIDMUS 24/26 MG TABLET 14
49. CILACAR 10 MG TABLET 15
50. CIPREMI 100 MG INJECTION 1
51. CLARIBID 500 MG TABLET 10
52. CLAVAM 500/125 MG TABLET 10
53. CLEXANE 40 MG INJECTION 0.4 ML
54. CLEXANE 60 MG INJECTION 0.6 ML
55. COBADEX CZS TABLET 15
56. CODISTAR 4/10 MG SYRUP 100 ML
57. COMBIFLAM 400/325 MG TABLET 20
58. CONCOR 5 MG TABLET 10
59. COREX DX 4/10 MG SYRUP 100 ML
60. CREMAFFIN PLUS SF 1.25 ML/3.75ML/3.33MG LIQUID 225 ML
61. CYPON 275/2 MG SYRUP 200 ML
62. CYRA D 30/20 MG TABLET SR 10
63. DALACIN C 300 MG CAPSULE 10
64. DECA DURABOLIN 50 MG INJECTION 1
65. DEFCORT 6 MG TABLET 10
66. DERIPHYLLIN 25.3/84.7 MG INJECTION 2 ML
67. DEROBIN 1.15/1.15/5.3 % OINTMENT 30 GM
68. DEXONA (VIAL) 4 MG INJECTION 2 ML
69. DEXORANGE 160 MG/0.5MG/7.5MCG SYRUP 200 ML
70. DOLO 650 MG TABLET 15
71. DOLONEX 20 MG TABLET DT 15
72. DOXINATE 10/10 MG TABLET 30
73. DOXT SL 100 MG/5BIU CAPSULE 10

74. DOXY 1 FORTE L DR 100 MG/5BIU CAPSULE 10
75. DULCOFLEX 5 MG TABLET 10
76. DUOLIN 3 1.25 MG/500MCG RESPULES 3 ML
77. DUPHASTON 10 MG TABLET 10
78. DYDROBOON 10 MG TABLET 10
79. DYNAPAR AQ 75 MG INJECTION 1 ML
80. EASY SIX PREFILLED SYRINGE 0.5 ML
81. ECOSPRIN AV 10/75 MG CAPSULE 15
82. ECOSPRIN GOLD 75/20/75 MG TABLET 15
83. ELAXIM 40 MG INJECTION 1
84. ELECTRAL SACHET 21.8 GM
85. ELIQUIS 2.5 MG TABLET 10
86. ELIQUIS 5 MG TABLET 10
87. ELTROXIN 100 MCG TABLET 120
88. ENTEROGERMINA 2 BIU ORAL SUSPENSION 5 ML
89. EXHEP 40 MG PREFILLED SYRINGE 0.4 ML
90. FABIFLU 200 MG TABLET 34
91. FABIFLU 400 MG TABLET 17
92. FABIFLU COPACK 800 MG TABLET 18
93. FARONEM 200 MG TABLET 10
94. FARONEM 300 MG TABLET ER 10
95. FORACORT 20/500 MCG RESPULES 2 ML
96. FORACORT 6/200 MCG ROTACAP 30
97. FORACORT 6/400 MCG ROTACAP 30
98. FORXIGA 10 MG TABLET 14
99. GABAPIN NT 400/10 MG TABLET 15
100. GALVUS 50 MG TABLET 15
101. GALVUS MET 50/1000 MG TABLET 15
102. GALVUS MET 50/500 MG TABLET 15
103. GEFTINAT 250 MG TABLET 30
104. GELUSIL MPS 250/50/250 MG LIQUID 200 ML
105. GEMCAL 500 MG/0.25MCG/7.5MG CAPSULE 15
106. GEMER 2/500 MG TABLET 10
107. GIBTULIO 25 MG TABLET 10
108. GLUCONORM-G 2/500 MG TABLET 15
109. GLYCOMET GP 1/500 MG TABLET 15
110. GLYCOMET GP 2/500 MG TABLET SR 15
111. GLYNASE MF 5/500 MG TABLET 10
112. GLYXAMBI 25/5 MG TABLET 10
113. GRILINCTUS 60/2.5/5/50 MG SYRUP 100 ML

114. GUDCEF 200 MG TABLET 10
115. GUDCEF CV 200/125 MG TABLET 10
116. HCQS 200 MG TABLET 15
117. HEXAXIM INJECTION 0.5 ML
118. HUCOG HP 5000 IU INJECTION 1 ML
119. HUMINSULIN 30/70 100 IU CARTRIDGE 3 ML
120. INFANRIX HEXA INJECTION 0.5 ML
121. ISTAMET 50/500 MG TABLET 15
122. IVABRAD 5 MG TABLET 15
123. IVERMECTOL NEW 12 MG TABLET 2
124. JALRA M 50/500 MG TABLET 15
125. JANUMET 50/1000 MG TABLET 15
126. JANUMET 50/500 MG TABLET 15
127. JANUVIA 100 MG TABLET 7
128. JARDIANCE 10 MG TABLET 10
129. JARDIANCE 25 MG TABLET 10
130. KABIMOL 1000 MG INFUSION 100 ML
131. KARVOL PLUS CAPSULE 10
132. KENACORT 40 MG INJECTION 1 ML
133. KETOROL 10 MG TABLET DT 15
134. KETOSTERIL TABLET 20
135. LANTUS 100 IU CARTRIDGE 3 ML
136. LANTUS SOLOSTAR 100 IU DISPOSABLE PEN 3 ML
137. LEVERA 500 MG TABLET 15
138. LEVIPIL 500 MG TABLET 10
139. LIBRAX 2.5/5 MG TABLET 20
140. LIMCEE CHEW ORANGE 500 MG TABLET 15
141. LIPAGLYN 4 MG TABLET 10
142. LMWX 40 MG INJECTION 0.4 ML
143. LOBATE GM NEO 0.05/0.5/2 % CREAM 15 GM
144. LONOPIN 40 MG INJECTION 0.4 ML
145. LOSAR 50 MG TABLET 15
146. LOSAR H 50/12.5 MG TABLET 15
147. MACBERY XT 50/1.25/4 MG SYRUP 100 ML
148. MAGNEX FORTE 1000/500 MG INJECTION 1
149. MANFORCE 100 MG TABLET 4
150. MANFORCE 50 MG TABLET 9
151. MAXTRA 5/2 MG SYRUP 60 ML
152. MEFTAL SPAS 10/250 MG TABLET 10
153. MEGALIS 20 MG TABLET 4

154. MEGANEURON OD PLUS 1500 MCG CAPSULE 10
155. MENACTRA INJECTION 0.5 ML
156. MERO 1000 MG INJECTION 1
157. MEROMAC 1000 MG INJECTION 1
158. MERONEM 1000 MG INJECTION 1
159. MEROZA 1000 MG INJECTION 1 ML
160. MIFEGEST KIT 200 MG/200MCG TABLET 1
161. MIKACIN 500 MG INJECTION 2 ML
162. MINIPRESS XL 5 MG TABLET XL 30
163. MIXTARD HM PENFILL 30/70 100 IU INJECTION 3 ML
164. MIXTARD HUMAN 30/70 40 IU INJECTION 10 ML
165. MIXTARD HUMAN 50/50 40 IU INJECTION 10 ML
166. MONOCEF 1000 MG INJECTION 5 ML
167. MONOCEF O 200 MG TABLET 10
168. MONOCEF SB 1000/500 MG INJECTION 1
169. MONTAIR LC 10/5 MG TABLET 15
170. MONTAZ 1000/125 MG INJECTION 1
171. MONTEK-LC 10/5 MG TABLET 10
172. MONTICOPE 10/5 MG TABLET 10
173. MOX 500 MG CAPSULE 15
174. MOX CV 500/125 MG TABLET 10
175. MOXCLAV 500/125 MG TABLET 10
176. MOXIKIND CV 500/125 MG TABLET 10
177. MUCAINE MINT 10/291/98 MG GEL 200 ML
178. MUCINAC SF ORANGE 600 MG TABLET 10
179. NEBICARD 5 MG TABLET 10
180. NEFROSAVE 150/500 MG TABLET 15
181. NEUROBION FORTE TABLET 30
182. NEXPRO 40 MG TABLET 15
183. NEXPRO RD 30/40 MG CAPSULE 10
184. NIKORAN 5 MG TABLET 20
185. NISE 100 MG TABLET 15
186. NITROCONTIN 2.6 MG TABLET CR 30
187. NOVOMIX 100 IU CARTRIDGE 3 ML
188. NOVOMIX 30/70 MG FLEXPEN 3 ML
189. NOVORAPID 100 IU CARTRIDGE 3 ML
190. NUROKIND LC 500 MG/1.5MG/1500MCG TABLET 15
191. NUROKIND PLUS RF 1500 MCG CAPSULE 10
192. O2 200/500 MG TABLET 10
193. OMEZ 20 MG CAPSULE 20

194. OMEZ D 30/20 MG CAPSULE SR 15
195. OMNIKACIN 500 MG INJECTION 2 ML
196. ONDERO 5 MG TABLET 10
197. ONDERO MET 2.5/500 MG TABLET 10
198. OROFER FCM INJECTION 10 ML
199. OROFER-XT 100/1.5 MG TABLET 10
200. OROFER-XT PLUS 30 MG/500MCG/500MCG SUSPENSION 200 ML
201. OTRIVIN OXY FAST RELIEF 0.05 % SPRAY 10 ML
202. OVRAL L 0.03/0.15 MG TABLET 21
203. OXRA 10 MG TABLET 14
204. PAN 40 MG TABLET 15
205. PAN D 30/40 MG CAPSULE 15
206. PANDERM PLUS PLUS 0.05/0.5/2 % CREAM 15 GM
207. PANTIN IV 40 MG INJECTION 10 ML
208. PANTOCID 40 MG TABLET 15
209. PANTOCID DSR 30/40 MG CAPSULE 15
210. PANTODAC 40 MG TABLET 15
211. PANTODAC DSR 30/40 MG CAPSULE 15
212. PANTOP 40 MG INJECTION 10 ML
213. PANTOP 40 MG TABLET 15
214. PANTOP D 10/20 MG CAPSULE 10
215. PANTOP D SR 30/40 MG CAPSULE SR 10
216. PHENSEDYL COUGH LINCTUS 4/10 MG SYRUP 100 ML
217. PIPZO 4000/500 MG INJECTION 10 ML
218. PRACTIN 4 MG TABLET 10
219. PREGA NEWS KIT 6
220. PREVENAR 13 INJECTION 0.5 ML
221. R.B TONE SYRUP 200 ML
222. RABLET-D 30/20 MG CAPSULE 10
223. RANTAC 150 MG TABLET 30
224. RAZO 20 MG TABLET 15
225. RAZO D 30/20 MG TABLET 15
226. REFRESH TEARS 0.5 % EYE DROPS 10 ML
227. REJUNEX-CD3 TABLET 10
228. REMDAC 100 MG INJECTION 1
229. ROSUVAS 10 MG TABLET 15
230. ROSUVAS 20 MG TABLET 10
231. RYZODEG 2.56/1.05 MG PENFILL 3 ML
232. SARIDON 250/50/150 MG TABLET 10

233. SEROFLO 50/250 MCG ROTACAP 30
234. SHELCAL 500 MG/250IU TABLET 15
235. SHELCAL XT 500 MG/2000IU/1500MCG/1MG/20MG TABLET 15
236. SILODAL 8 MG TABLET 10
237. SILODAL D 8/0.5 MG TABLET 10
238. SINAREST 125/5/1 MG SYRUP 60 ML
239. SINAREST NEW 500/10/2 MG TABLET 10
240. SINAREST NEW 500/10/2 MG TABLET 15
241. SKINLITE 2/0.1/0.025 % CREAM 25 GM
242. SOMPRAZ D 30/40 MG CAPSULE 15
243. SPASMO PROXYVON PLUS 10/325/50 MG CAPSULE 8
244. SPEGRA 50/200/25 MG TABLET 30
245. STAMLO 5 MG TABLET 30
246. STAMLO BETA 50/5 MG TABLET 15
247. STEMETIL 5 MG TABLET MD 15
248. SUCRAFIL O 1000/20 MG GEL 200 ML
249. SUMO 100/325 MG TABLET 15
250. SUMO L IV 1000 MG INFUSION 100 ML
251. SUPRADYN TABLET 15
252. SYNFLORIX INJECTION 1
253. T BACT 2 % OINTMENT 15 GM
254. T BACT 2 % OINTMENT 5 GM
255. TARGOCID 400 MG INJECTION 1 ML
256. TAXIM O 200 MG TABLET 10
257. TAZOMAC 4000/500 MG INJECTION 2 ML
258. TELEKAST-L 10/5 MG TABLET 15
259. TELMA 40 MG TABLET 30
260. TELMA AM 40/5 MG TABLET 15
261. TELMA H 40/12.5 MG TABLET 15
262. TELMIKIND 40 MG TABLET 10
263. TELMIKIND AM 40/5 MG TABLET 10
264. TELMIKIND H 40/12.5 MG TABLET 10
265. THROMBOPHOB OINTMENT 20 GM
266. THYRONORM 100 MCG TABLET 120
267. THYRONORM 25 MCG TABLET 120
268. THYRONORM 50 MCG TABLET 120
269. TOSSEX NEW 4/10 MG SYRUP 100 ML
270. TRAJENTA 5 MG TABLET 10
271. TRESIBA FLEXTOUCH 100 IU DISPOSABLE PEN 3 ML
272. TUSQ DX 5/2/15 MG SYRUP 100 ML

273. UDILIV 150 MG TABLET 15
274. UDILIV 300 MG TABLET 15
275. ULTRACET 325/37.5 MG TABLET 15
276. UNIENZYME TABLET 15
277. UNWANTED 72 1.5 MG TABLET 1
278. UNWANTED KIT 200 MG/200MCG TABLET 1
279. UPRISE D3 60000 IU CAPSULE 8
280. URIMAX 0.4 MG CAPSULE 20
281. URIMAX D 0.4/0.5 MG TABLET 15
282. URSOCOL 300 MG TABLET 15
283. VARILRIX INJECTION 0.5 ML
284. VELOZ D 30/20 MG CAPSULE SR 10
285. VELPANAT 400/100 MG TABLET 28
286. VERTIN 16 MG TABLET 15
287. VOLINI 1.16 % SPRAY 40 GM
288. VORIER 200 MG TABLET 4
289. VOVERAN SR 100 MG TABLET SR 15
290. VYMADA 24/26 MG TABLET 14
291. WYSOLONE 10 MG TABLET DT 15
292. WYSOLONE 5 MG TABLET DT 15
293. XONE 1000 MG INJECTION 5 ML
294. ZAVICEFTA 2000/500 MG VIAL 10 ML
295. ZEDEX 4/5/50 MG SYRUP 100 ML
296. ZERODOL P 100/325 MG TABLET 10
297. ZERODOL SP 100/325/15 MG TABLET 10
298. ZIFI 200 MG TABLET 10
299. ZORYL-M 2/500 MG TABLET 20
300. ZOSTUM 1000/500 MG INJECTION 1

Schedule K Drugs: According to the Rule 123 of Drugs Rules, the drugs specified in Schedule K are exempted from the provisions of Chapter IV of the Drugs and Cosmetics Act, 1940 (i.e rules prescribed for manufacture, sale and distribution of drugs) with certain conditions. Some of these drugs are sold and prescribed under some specific situations as defined under the list of Schedule K. List of Schedule K drugs includes (as updated till 2023):

1. Drugs Labelled as 'Not for medicinal Use'
2. Omitted
    2A. Quinine and other antimalarial drugs.
3. Omitted

4. Omitted
5. Drugs supplied by a Allopathic Doctor to own patient or any prescription drugs on conditions that the doctor is not keeping an open shop, not selling across counter, engaged in import, manufacture, distribution or sale of drugs in India.
    5A. Drugs supplied by a hospital or dispensary maintained or supported by Government or local body.
    5B. Whole Human Blood IP and / or its components stored for transfusion.
6. Omitted
7. Quinine sulphate
8. Omitted
9. Magnesium sulphate
10. Substances used both as articles of food as well as drugs like all condensed or powdered milk (pure, skimmed or malted, fortified with vitamins and minerals), or farex, oats, and all other similar cereal preparations whether fortified with vitamins or otherwise excepting those for parenteral use, virol, bovril, chicken essence and all other similar predigested foods, ginger, pepper, cumin, cinnamon and all other similar spices and condiments.
11. Omitted
12. Substances intended to be used for destruction of vermin or insects which cause disease in human beings or animals, viz. Insecticides and Disinfectants.
13. Household remedies like: Aspirin tablets, Paracetamol Tablets, Analgesic Balms, Antacid preparations, Gripe Water for use of infants, Inhalers containing drugs for treatment of cold and nasal congestion, Syrups/lozenges/pills/tablets for cough, Liniments for external use, Skin ointments and ointments for burns, Absorbent cotton wool, bandages, absorbent guaze and adhesive plaster, Castor Oil, liquid Paraffin, Epsom Salt, Eucalyptus Oil, Tincture Iodine, Tincture Benzoin Co. and Mercurochrome in containers not exceeding 100 ml, Tablets of Quinine Sulphate I.P., Tablets of Iodochlorohydroxy quinoline-250 mg.
14. Mechanical Contraceptives.
    14A. Vaginal contraceptive pessaries containing Nonoxynol.
15. Chemical contraceptive having the following composition per tablet:
    - DL-Norgestrel-0.30 mg + Ethinyl Estradiol-0.03 mg,
    - Levonorgestrel-0.15 mg + Ethinyl Estradiol-0.03 mg,

- Centchroman-30 mg,
- Desogestrel-0.15 mg + Ethinyl Estradiol 0.03 mg,
- Levonorgestrel-0.1 mg + Ethinyl Estradiol 0.02 mg.

16. Omitted.
17. Ophthalmic ointments of the Tetracycline group of drugs.
18. Omitted.
19. Hair Fixers, namely mucilaginous preparations containing gums, used by men for fixing beard.
20. Radio Pharmaceuticals.
21. Tablets of Chloroquine Salts.
22. Sales from restaurant cars of trains and from coastal ships of household remedies, which do not require the supervision of a qualified person for their sale.
23. Drugs supplied by multipurpose workers attached to Primary Health Centres/Sub- Centres, Community Health Volunteers under the Rural Health Scheme, Nurses, Auxiliary Nurses, Midwives, Lady Health Visitors attached to Urban Family Welfare Centres/Primary Health Centres/Sub Centres and Anganwadi Workers.
24. Homeopathic medicines supplied by a registered Homoeopathic Doctor to own patient.
25. Preparations applied to the human body for the purpose of repelling insects like mosquitoes.
26. Medicated Dressing and Bandages for First Aid.
27. Oral Rehydration Salts manufactured as per the following formula as Sodium chloride 3.5 g/litre, Trisodium citrate dehydrate 2.9 g/litre, Potassium Chloride 1.5 g/ litre. May be replaced by Sodium bicarbonate (Sodium hydrogen Carbonate) 2.5 g/ litre, when citrate salt is not available.
28. White or Yellow Petroleum Jelly I.P. (Non-perfumed).
29. Morphine Tablets
30. Whole Human Blood collected and transfused by Centres run by Armed Forces Medical Services in border areas, small mid-zonal hospitals including peripheral hospitals, Field Ambulances, Mobile medical units and other field medical units including blood supply units in border, sensitive and field areas.
31. Homeopathic Medicines.
32. First Aid kit supplied along with motor vehicle by the manufacturer or its distributors at the time of first sale of vehicle.
33. Nicotine gum and Lozenges containing upto 2 mg of nicotine.

34. Production of Oxygen 93% USP produced from air by the molecular sieve process, by a hospital or Medical Institute for their captive consumption.
35. Homoeopathic hair oils having active ingredients up to 3X potency only.
36. Custom made devices.
37. Zinc sulphate tablets and oral solutions having 10 and 20 mg of elemental zinc.
38. Sterile solutions intended for parenteral administration with 100 ml in one container manufactured for export only.
39. Antiseptic liquid for household use.

Schedule E1 Drugs: As per Rule 161(2) of the Drugs Rules, the list of poisonous substances under the Ayurvedic (including Siddha) and Unani Systems of Medicine is mentioned in Schedule E(1) and required to be taken under medical supervision only. In nut shell, these drugs should be consumed only under proper medical supervision and with prescription inorder to avoid the risks of toxicity. Hence, a Ayurvedic, Siddha or Unani registered medical practitioner's prescription is required for its sale to the patient.

A. AYURVEDIC SYSTEM
  I. Drugs of vegetable origin:
     1. Ahipena (except seeds) - *Papaver somniferum*
     2. Arka - *Calotropis procera*
     3. Bhallataka - *Semecarpus anacardium*
     4. Bhanga (except seeds) - *Cannabis sativa*
     5. Danti - *Baliospermum montanum*
     6. Dhattura - *Datura metal*
     7. Gunja (seed) - *Abrus precatorium*
     8. Jaipala (seed) - *Croton tiglium*
     9. Karaveera - *Rerium indicum*
     10. Langali - *Gloriosa superba*
     11. Parasika Yavani - *Hyoscyamus niger*
     12. Vatsanabha - *Acontium chasmanthum*
         Vishamushti - *Strychnox nuxvomica*
     13. Shringivisha - *Acontium chasmanthum*

  II. Drugs of Animal Origin:
     14. Sarpa Visha - Snake poison

III. Drugs of Mineral Origin:
   15. Gauripashana - Arsenic
   16. Hartala - Arseno sulphide
   17. Manahashila - Arseno sulphide
   18. Parada/Parad - Mercury
   19. Rasa Karpura - Hydrargyri subchloridum
   20. Tuttha - Copper sulphate
   21. Hingula - Cinnabar

B. SIDDHA SYSTEM
   1. Abini - *Papaver somniferum*
   2. Alari - *Nerium indicum*
   3. Attru thummatti - *Citrullus colocynthis*
   4. Umathai - *Datura stramonium*
   5. Etti - *Stychnos nux vomica*
   6. Ganja (except seed) - *Cannabis sativa*
   7. Kalappaki Kizahangu - *Glorisa superba*
   8. Kodikkalli (exempted for external use) - *Euphorbia tirucalli*
   9. Kattu Thumatti - *Cucumis trigonus*
   10. Kunri (except root) - *Arbus precatorius*
   11. Cheramkottai - *Semecarpus anacardium*
   12. Thillai - *Exoecoria agallocha*
   13. Nabi - *Aconitum ferox*
   14. Nervalam - *Croton tiglium*
   15. Pugaielai - *Nicotiana tabacum*
   16. Mancevikkalli - *Euphorbia*

C. UNANI SYSTEM
   I. Drugs of vegetable origin:
   1. Afiyun (except seed) - *Papaver somniferum*
   2. Bazrul banj - *Hyoscyamus niger*
   3. Bish - *Aconitum chasmanthum Stapf ex Holmes*
   4. Bhang - *Cannabis sativa*
   5. Charas - *Cannabis sativa*
   6. Dhatura/Datura seeds - *Datura metal*
   7. Kuchla - *Strychnos nuxvomica*
   8. Shokran - *Conium maculatum*

   II. Drugs of Animal origin:
   1. Sanp (head) - Snake (head).

2. Telni makkhi - *Mylabris cichori, Mylabaris pustulata, Mylabris macilenta*

III. <u>Drugs of Mineral origin</u>:
1. Darchikna - *Hydrargryi perchloridum*
2. Hira - *Diamond*
3. Ras Kapoor - *Hydrargryi Subchloridum (calomel)*
4. Shingruf - *Hydrargryi bisulphuratum*
5. Zangar - *Cupri subacetas*
6. Sammul-Far - *(Abyaz, Asfar, Aswad and Ahmar) (white, yellow, black and red, Arsenic)*
7. Tootiya - *Copper Sulphate*
8. Para - *Hydrargyrum*
9. Hartal - *Arsenic trisulphide (yellow)*

CHAPTER 4

Allopathic Drugs Sale Rule

Introduction

In India, for both retail and wholesale medicine business i.e. sale or resale of allopathic drugs (prescription or non-prescription) an individual or firm requires a valid 'Drug Sale License' issued by the State Licensing Authority (SLA), State Drug Control Department. Besides this, GST registration, Trade Licenses and Shop & Establishment registration, and FSSAI registration (if selling food products) are also required as per State Licensing Authority to operate a retail or wholesale pharmacy.

Drug Sale License

A Drug Sale License is granted by the State Licensing Authority in 4 types:

- Retail Sale Drug License (RSDL) - Form 20 and 21 intended for sale to patient or end customers (B2C).
- Wholesale Drug License (WSDL) - Form 20B and 21B intended for resale or wholesale purpose (B2B).
- Combined Retail and Wholesale Drug License - Form 20, 21, 20B and 21B intended for both retail and resale purpose (B2C + B2B).
- Restricted License (for Household remedies) - Form 20A and 21A intended for sale to patient or end customer (B2C).

A drug sale license is location or premise specific, so if allopathic drugs are sold, stocked or distributed from more than one place, the licensee shall have a separate drug sale license for that particular premise/location. Hence, the thumb rule of 'ONE PREMISE - ONE DRUG SALE LICENSE' always prevail for the drug business.

Pre-Licensing Requirements

An applicant shall follow the below procedures to obtain a fresh Retail & Wholesale Drug license:

- Stage 1: (Online Application) - The Applicant has to apply online to the State Licensing Authority i.e. Senior Drug Control Officer cum-Licensing Authority of the Zone. The user can pay application fees via online mode through Net Banking/Debit Card/Credit Card or State Government Treasury challan which can be downloaded and uploaded while the online application. The applicant has to make an application in the requisite Form viz 19, 19A,19B, 19AA. The details of Forms and fees is given in the fee chart in the below table.

- Stage 2: (Premise Inspection) - The Application is scrutinized and premises is inspected by DCO of the Concerned District and the report is forwarded by DCO along with his recommendation to SDCO of the Zone and during inspection DCO should verify all facilities provided and documents uploaded by the applicant.

- Stage 3: (Grant of License) - If all the conditions as prescribed by the Drugs and Cosmetics Act and Rules thereunder are found complied, the sale drug licence is granted by SDCO-cum-Licensing Authority (Retail/wholesale) and applicant gets information through SMS/email.

Pre-Licensing Documents

An applicant has to submit documents during online application process including:

- Covering letter to be addressed to the Drugs Controller and State Licensing Authority, Drugs Control Department.
- Requisite duly signed Application Form (Form viz 19, 19A,19B, 19AA).
- Receipt for the fees of Rs. 3000/- paid or challan (for retail or wholesale), as the case may be or their attested copies.
- Sketch plan with actual dimensions, surrounding and signature of proprietor / partner / director of the proposed firm to be applied in 3 copies.
- Documents viz. rent receipt, sub lease agreement, rent agreement, purchase documents or its attested copies showing lawful possession of the premises.

- Documents relating to the constitution of the firm viz. Partnership-deed, memorandum and article of association etc. and their affidavits w.r.t. non conviction.
- Full particulars of the registered pharmacist (in case of retail pharmacy) along with copies of their educational qualification, experience and registration certificates from particular State Pharmacy Council.
- Full particulars of the competent person (in case of wholesale pharmacy) along with copies of their educational qualification, experience certificates from previous firm.
- Full name of the proprietor or the partners, as the case may be, shall be provided in the application.
- In case of private or public limited concerns, full name of the Directors who sign the application and the authorized signatory, if any, shall be provided in the application.
- Purchase voucher of Refrigerator/Deep freezer (For Vaccines/Sera).
- Purchase voucher of AC (applicable in some states).
- Affidavit of Biomedical waste by authorized signatory (applicable in some states).
- Affidavit of authorized signatory (registered pharmacist, competent person, directors etc.).
- Copy of resolution of Board of Directors for Authorized Signatory.

NOTE: *After receipt application alongwith required documents, the same is forwarded to DCO (Drug Control Officer) of the concerned District for scrutiny and inspection.*

Infrastructure requirement

- For Retail Sale Drug License (RSDL) Form 20, 21 - Required area of premises should be minimum of 10 sq. mt. with min. 8'2" height. Premises should be brick built, plastered floor cemented.
- For Wholesale Drug License (WSDL) Form 20B, 21B - Required area of premises should be minimum of 10 sq. mt. with min. 8'2" height. Premises should be brick built, plastered floor cemented.
- For Retail and Wholesale Combined Drug Sale License (in same premise) - Required area of premises should be minimum of 15 sq.

mt. with min. 8'2" height. Premises should be brick built, plastered floor cemented.

Qualified Person

Following documents of a 'Registered Pharmacist - RP' or 'Competent Person - CP' are required during the process of a drug sale license application:

1. <u>For Retail Sale Drug License (RSDL)</u> - Services of Registered Pharmacist (RP) is mandatory for RSDL with below documents:
   - Affidavit from the Registered Pharmacist,
   - Proof of qualification i.e. final degree certificate/provisional certificate with mark sheets,
   - Valid pharmacist registration certificate (to be issued from that state pharmacy council where drug sale license has been applied and drug business will be operated),
   - Appointment Letter and Bio-data,
   - Identity proof (PAN and Adhar card copy).

2. <u>For Wholesale Drug License (WSDL)</u> - Services of Competent Person (CP) is mandatory for WSDL whose qualification can be:
   a) Graduate with min. 1 year experience in sale of allopathic drugs or,
   b) Registered Pharmacist (RP) or,
   c) Matriculation with min. 4 years experience in purchase and sale of allopathic drugs .

   Following documents of Competent Person are required for the application of wholesale drug license:
   - Affidavit from the Competent Person,
   - Proof of qualification i.e. final degree certificate/provisional certificate with mark sheets,
   - Experience Certificate (mandatory for non-registered pharmacist),
   - Pharmacist registration certificate - In case CP is a registered pharmacist, then pharmacist registration certificate is required which shall be issued from that state pharmacy council where

drug sale license has been applied and drug business will be operated,
- Appointment Letter and Bio-data
- Identity proof (PAN and Aadhar card copy)

NOTE: *Documents of a qualified person required during the drug sale license application may vary from state to state licensing authority. Hence it is advisable to check the particular state licensing authority drug control department for documents requirements.*

Storage facility

1. <u>For Retail Sale Drug License (RSDL)</u> - Purchase bills of A/C and refrigerator along with Working condition/Installation Certificate is also required by some states.
2. <u>For Wholesale Drug License (WSDL)</u> - Purchase bills of A/C and refrigerator along with Working condition/Installation Certificate is also required by some states.   In case the licensee has also installed a 'Cold Room Walking Chiller' it shall have a temperature monitoring logger system installed to monitor daily temperature to be maintained between +2°C to +8°C temperature.

NOTE: *As a Good Distribution Practice (GDP) of pharmaceutical goods it is advisable to maintain room temperature below 25 degrees celsius. Also, temperature logger devices shall be installed in prominent place to capture the daily temperature and humidity (RH) of the drug licensed premise. This will help to maintain and track the room temperature thereby maintaining efficacy and quality of the stocked medicines making it safe and efficient to be consumed by the patient.*

Equipements, Furniture and Facilities

For both Retail and Wholesale Drug License storage facilities racks, Refrigerator, Proper lightning, Ventilation, A/C (optional), Fans, and Cupboard/Drawer with lock & key has to be provided. Besides this, sitting arrangements for the pharmacist and competent persons shall be provided with computer system for billing, and a printer for tax invoice printing.

Application Fees

- Retail Sale Drug License - For a Fresh or Renewal of Retail License total fee prescribed is Rs. 3000/- (Rs. 1500 for Form 20 and Rs. 1500 for Form 21).
- Wholesale Drug License - For a Fresh or Renewal of Wholesale License total fee prescribed is Rs. 3000/- (Rs. 1500 for Form 20B and Rs. 1500 for Form 21B).
- Combined Retail and Wholesale Drug License - For a Fresh or Renewal of Combined Retail and Wholesale License total fee prescribed is Rs. 6000/- (Rs. 1500 for Form 20, Rs. 1500 for Form 21, Rs. 1500 for Form 20B and Rs. 1500 for Form 21B).
- Retail Sale of Schedule X drugs - For a Fresh or Renewal of Retail License (Form 20F) total fee prescribed is Rs. 500.
- Wholesale of Schedule X drugs - For Fresh or Renewal of Wholesale License (Form 20G) total fee prescribed is Rs. 500.
- Combined Retail and Wholesale of Schedule X drugs - For Fresh or Renewal of Combined License (Form 20F and 20G) total fee prescribed is Rs. 1000.
- Restricted License - For Fresh or Renewal of Restricted License (Form 20A and 21A) total fee prescribed is Rs. 1000.

NOTE: *The license in Form 20F or 20G for sale of Schedule X drugs shall be applied separately. Never apply for these licenses with licenses in Form 20, 21, 20B, 21B.*

Type of Drug Sale License with prescribed fees

Application Form	Drug Sale License	License Type	Fresh License	Renewal License	Duplicate copy fees
19	Form 20	Retail Allopathy	Rs. 1500	Rs. 1500	Rs. 150
19	Form 21	Retail Allopathy	Rs. 1500	Rs. 1500	Rs. 150
19	Form 20B	Wholesale Allopathy	Rs. 1500	Rs. 1500	Rs. 150
19	Form 21B	Wholesale Allopathy	Rs. 1500	Rs. 1500	Rs. 150
19A	Form 20A	Retail Restricted	Rs. 500	Rs. 500	Rs. 150
19A	Form 21A	Retail Restricted	Rs. 500	Rs. 500	Rs. 150
19A*	Form 20A*	Retail Restricted	Rs. 10	Rs. 10	Rs. 2
19A*	Form 21A*	Retail Restricted	Rs. 10	Rs. 10	Rs. 2
19AA	Form 20BB	Vehicle	Rs. 500	Rs. 500	Rs. 150
19AA	Form 21BB	Vehicle	Rs. 500	Rs. 500	Rs. 150
19C	Form 20F	Retail - Schedule X	Rs. 500	Rs. 500	Rs. 150
19C	Form 20G	Wholesale - Schedule X	Rs. 500	Rs. 500	Rs. 150

In case of itinerant vendors or applicants who desire to establish a shop in town or village having population 5000 or less.

Conditions for change in the licensed premise

- <u>Change in Constitution</u>: If the firm changes from proprietorship to partnership including Limited Liability Partnership or vice versa or from a Private to a Public company, or from a Public to a Private company it shall be treated as 'change in constitution'. If any change in constitution takes place a new sale drug license is to be obtained within three months of the said change in constitution. The fees for Change in Constitution is same as that of Fresh License.

- <u>Change in Premise or Address</u>: When there is a change in address of the drug licensed premises, the drug sale license for the old premises has to be surrendered, and the drug business owner has to apply for a new drug sale licence for the new proposed premises. If any change in address takes place a new sale drug license is to be obtained within three months of the said change. The fees for Change in premise or address is same as that of Fresh License.

- <u>Change in Qualified Person</u>: When there is any change in qualified person like resignation or new joining of a registered pharmacist (RP) or competent person (CP), the licensee shall inform the State Licensing Authority (SLA) with an application for endorsement or removal of his name (as the case may be) within one month of time. There is no fee prescribed for change in Qualified Person.

- <u>Addition or Reduction in area</u>: When there is any reduction or addition in the existing approved drug licensed area then the licensee needs to inform to the State Licensing Authority (SLA) about the proposed change with application form, drug license copy, existing maplayout and proposed changes to be made in maplayout. There is no fee prescribed for addition or reduction in the area of the same licensed premise.

Post-Licensing Requirements for a Retail Pharmacy

If a Retail Pharmacy already possess a Allopathic Retail Sale Drug License (Form 20 & 21) then, there is no requirement for having a separate Homeopathic Retail Sale Drug License (Form 20C) or Medical Device Registration Certificate (Form MD 42). In a nutshell, if a retail pharmacy already possess a RSDL (i.e. Form 20 & 21) the entity can continue his retail business of allopathic drugs, homeopathic drugs and medical devices on the same RSDL under supervision of the same endorsed Registered Pharmacist (RP).

After receiving a Retail Sale Drug License (RSDL - Form 20 & 21) a retail pharmacy should adhere to the following compliances:

- Signboard at entry point - Sign board with licensee name, complete address with pin code, and GST number (if any) with word 'Chemist and Druggist' shall be displayed at the entry point of the firm (in case a drug licensee employs a registered pharmacist). All details on the signboard should be exactly the same as mentioned in the drug sale license.
- Retail Sale Drug License - An original valid drug sale license (Form 20 & 21) shall be displayed at a prominent place. A drug sale license shall be renewed from time to time by the licensee every 5 years utill and unless suspended or canceled by the State Licensing Authority.
- FSSAI registration/license - If a retailer is involved in sale of any food supplements it shall display the FFSAI registration/license at the prominent place.
- Trade license and Shop & Establishment - A retailer should also obtain a trade license and a shop and establishment registration as per the state specific requirements. Example in West Bengal Trade License/Trade Enlistment Certificate with nature of trade of medicine is mandatory.
- Endorsed Registrered Pharmacist documents - All the sale, purchase and dispensation of the drugs shall be conducted under the personal supervision of the registered pharmacist only as he is only the custodian of overall responsibility in a pharmacy. No medicine shall be dispensed in case the endorsed registered pharmacist is not available or absent. Registration certificate for the pharmacist issued from the state pharmacy council shall be displayed at the prominent place. A retailer shall keep copies of all the documents of the endorsed registered pharmacist, i.e., registration certificate, qualification certificates, and address proof. Besides this, a retailer shall also maintain copies of all the documents regarding the change of endorsed registered pharmacist (RP). Application to the Drug Department with the details and dates of relieving the previously endorsed RP and joining the new RP, copy of pharmacist registration certificate, qualification certificates, address proof. Daily attendance record/register of the registered pharmacist shall be maintained in the licensed premise.

- <u>Purchase record</u> - The purchase invoice copy shall be maintained properly in a chronological order for minimum 2 years. Purchase record or invoice shall have the following details:
    (a) date of purchase
    (b) his name, address and drug license number
    (c) name of drug, quantity and batch number
    (d) name of manufacturer.

  A retailer shall always purchase the drugs from an authorized source having a valid Wholesale Drug License. The purchase order to the wholesaler / distributor on a signed written format shall have name, quantity and company name of the drug. While receiving the drugs orders in a retail registered pharmacist shall verify and match the quantity, batch no., expiry, name of company of purchased drug with received purchase invoice.

- <u>Sales record</u> - In a Retail Pharmacy a Competent Person (CP) is not authorized to sign bills/invoices. Only the endorsed Registered Pharmacist (RP) whose name is endorsed in the Retail Sale Drug License (RSDL) is authorized to sign it. The sales invoice copy shall be maintained properly in a chronological order for a minimum of 2 years. Sales record or invoice shall have the following details:

  (a) serial number of entry
  (b) date of supply
  (c) name and address of the prescriber/doctor
  (d) name and address of patient
  (e) name of drug and quantities
  (f) name of manufacturer, batch number and date of expiry
  (g) signature of the endorsed Registered Pharmacist (RP) by or under whose supervision the medicine was supplied.

- <u>Schedule X drug dispensing</u> - In the case of substances specified in Schedule X, the prescriptions shall be in duplicate, one copy of which shall be retained by the licensee for a period of 2 years.

- <u>Schedule H1 drug dispensing</u> - In the case of substance specified in Schedule H1, the Schedule H1 register/record shall be maintained by the retailer for minimum 3 years with details of name & address of doctor, name of patient, name and quantity of drug supplied.

- <u>Form 35</u> - The licensee shall maintain an Inspection Book in Form 35 to enable an Inspector to record his impressions and the defects noticed. This form can be procured from the State Drug Control Department branch on payment of prescribed fees.

- Seperate area for stocking Expired/Damaged drugs - All the expired/damaged drugs shall be stored separately from the trade stocks and all such drugs shall be kept in sepearte packages or cartons, the top of which shall display prominently, the words "Not for sale".
- Separate area for stocking Homeopathic drugs - All homeopathic drugs shall be kept separated from the allopathic drugs stocks and on the rack "Homeopathic medicines" shall be written.
- Separate area for stocking ASU (ayurvedic, siddha, unani) drugs - All ASU drugs shall be kept separated from the allopathic and homeopathic drugs stocks and on the rack "Ayurvedic, Siddha and Unani drugs" shall be written.
- Separate area for stocking Medical Devices - All medical devices shall be kept separated from the allopathic and homeopathic drugs stocks and on the rack "Medical Devices" shall be written.
- Separate area for stocking Veterinary drugs - The medicines for treatment of animals kept in a retail shop or premises shall be labeled with the words 'Not for human use for treatment of animals only' and shall be stored in a cupboard or drawer reserved solely for the storage of veterinary drugs, or in a part of the premises separated from the remainder of the premises.
- Prescription to be dispensed - Before dispensation an endorsed registered pharmacist shall check the prescription with the following details:

(a) Patient's name and address,
(b) Total medicine quantity and dose,
(c) Date of appointment
(d) Doctor's name, address, qualification, registration number and signature,
(e) Name and address of the pharmacy and date of medicine dispensation

A Pharmacist should never substitute the branded medicine mentioned on the RMPs prescription. In case only the generic name of the medicine is mentioned on the prescription then the pharmacist is authorized to substitute it with the same prescribed composition, strength and variant along with the patient's consent. The prescription must not be dispensed more than once unless the prescriber has stated thereon that it may be dispensed more than once. If the prescription contains a direction that it may be dispensed a stated number of times or at stated intervals it must not be dispensed otherwise than in accordance with the directions.

- Refrigerator - A retailer shall maintain the purchase record of the refrigerator. For storage of cold chain medicines a temperature range between +2 to +8 degree celsius is required for which a refrigerator shall be in working conditions and shall never be kept OFF. In case of electricity shortage or power failure an electricity power back-up shall be available to ensure that the refrigerator is not OFF and cold chain medicines' qfuality and efficacy does not get impacted due to temperature breach. Ensure no food articles, drinking water and oily injections e.g. Progesterone, Nandrolone, Decanoate etc. shall be stored inside the refrigerator.

- 'Physician sample' and 'Hospital supply drugs not for sale' - A pharmacy shall not stock and sell drugs with labels of 'Physician samples not for sale' and 'Hospital supply drugs not for sale'.

- Sale of Anti TB Drugs - Any Pharmacies involved in sale of Anti TB drugs needs to share patient details in Annexure III, a notification format provided in the GoI mandate to capture relevant patient details (including name, age, gender, GoI ID, address, phone number, date of TB diagnosis, date of treatment initiation, date of prescription, name and contact of treating doctor, date of dispensing of medicines, number of days for which medicines dispensed and other details such as reporting pharmacy contact details). Pharmacies should also fills details and submit drugs, patient and pharmacy details online on the Nikshay portal (https://www.nikshay.in/) a web based online web enabled patient management system for TB control under the National Tuberculosis Elimination Programme (NTEP). This portal is developed and maintained by the Central TB Division (CTD), Ministry of Health and Family Welfare, Government of India. Anti TB drugs include Schedule H1 drugs namely: Ethambutol, Ethionamide, Isoniazid, Levofloxacin, Moxifloxacin, Pyrazinamide, Rifabutin and Rifampicin.

NOTE: All registers and records maintained under these Rules shall be preserved for a period of not less than two years from the date of the last entry therein.

Post-Licensing Requirements for a Wholesale Pharmacy

For wholesale business of drugs an entity or individual requires a Wholesale Drug Sale License (WSDL) i.e. Form 20B & 21B. A Competent Person (CP) is mandatorily required under whose supervision all the wholesale business of drugs shall be carried out. After receiving a Wholesale Drug License (WSDL) the licensee should follow below important rules:

- <u>Signboard at entry point</u> - Sign board with licensee name, complete address with pin code, and GST number (if any) shall be displayed at the entry point of the firm.
- <u>Wholesale Drug License</u> - A valid drug sale license (Form 20B & 21B) shall be displayed at a prominent place. A drug sale license shall be renewed from time to time by the licensee every 5 years utill and unless suspended or canceled by the State Licensing Authority.
- <u>FSSAI registration/license</u> - If a wholesaler is involved in sale of any food supplements or articles it shall display the FSSAI registration/license at the prominent place.
- <u>Trade license and Shop & Establishment</u> - A wholesaler should also obtain a trade license and a shop and establishment registration as per the state specific requirements. Example in West Bengal Trade License/Trade Enlistment Certificate with nature of trade of medicine is mandatory.
- <u>Competent Person documents</u> - All the sale and purchase of the drugs shall be conducted under the personal supervision of the Competent Person (CP) only. No drugs shall be sold or purchased in case the endorsed Competent Person is not available or absent. In case the Competent Person (CP) is a Registered Pharmacist (RP) then his/her registration certificate issued from the state pharmacy council shall also be displayed at the prominent place. A wholesaler shall keep copies of all the documents of the Competent Person like qualification certificates, experience certificates (in case of non-pharmacist) and address proof. Besides this, a wholesaler shall also maintain copies of all the documents regarding the change of Competent Person (if any) like application to the Drug Department with the details and dates of relieving the previous CP and joining

of the new CP, copy of qualification certificates, experience certificates and address proof. Daily attendance record/register of the CP shall be maintained in the licensed premise.

- <u>Purchase record</u> - All the purchase records/invoices intended for resale shall be maintained by the wholesaler and such records shall show the following particulars, namely:

(a) date of purchase

(b) name, address and drug license number held by entity from whom purchased

(c) name of drug, quantity and batch number

(d) name of manufacturer.

Purchase bills/invoices shall be serially numbered by the wholesaler and maintained by him in a chronological order.

- <u>Sales record</u> - In a wholesale pharmacy a Competent Person (CP) is authorized to sign all the sales bills/invoices. All the sales record/invoices shall be maintained by the wholesaler and such records shall show the following particulars, namely:

(a) his name, address, drug license number of wholesaler

(b) date of sale

(c) name, address, drug license number of the licensee to whom sold

(d) name of drug, quantity and batch number

(e) name of manufacturer

(f) signature of competent person (CP) under whose supervision the sale was effected.

Duplicate bills shall be preserved as records for a period of 3 years from the date of the sale of the drug.

- <u>Form 35</u> - The licensee shall maintain an Inspection Book in Form 35 to enable an Inspector to record his impressions and the defects noticed. This form can be procured from the State Drug Control Department branch on payment of prescribed fees.

- <u>Separate area for stocking Expired/Damaged drugs</u> - All the expired/damaged drugs shall be stored separately from the trade stocks and all such drugs shall be kept in packages or cartons, the top of which shall display prominently, the words "Not for sale".

- <u>Separate area and sale license for stocking Homeopathic drugs</u> - A separate area and a fresh homeopathic wholesale drug license i.e. Form 20D shall be sought for wholesale business of homeopathic medicines.

- Separate area for stocking Veterinary drugs - The medicines for treatment of animals kept in a retail shop or premises shall be labeled with the words 'Not for human use for treatment of animals only' and shall be stored in a cupboard or drawer reserved solely for the storage of veterinary drugs, or in a part of the premises separated from the remainder of the premises.
- Refrigerator - A wholesaler shall maintain the purchase record of the refrigerator. For storage of cold chain medicines it requires a temperature range between +2 to +8 degree celsius for which a refrigerator shall be in working conditions and shall never be kept OFF. In case of electricity shortage or power failure an electricity power back-up shall be available to ensure that the refrigerator is not OFF and cold chain medicines' quality and efficacy does not get impacted due to temperature breach. Ensure no food articles, drinking water and oily injections e.g. Progesterone, Nandrolone, Decanoate etc. shall be stored inside the refrigerator. If a wholesaler has a cold room an alarm shall be installed to detect any temperature deviation from a range of +2 to +8 degree celsius.
- 'Physician sample' and 'Hospital supply drugs not for sale' - A wholesaler shall not stock and sell drugs with label of 'Physician samples not for sale' and 'Hospital supply drugs not for sale'.

CHAPTER 5

Homeopathic Medicines and Sale Rules

Historical Background of Homeopathy

The word 'Homeopathy' is made up of two Greek words namely '*Homois*' (means similar) and '*Pathos*' (means suffering). In 19th century Homeopathy started developing scientifically and the credit goes to the German physician, Dr. Samuel Hahnemann (1755-1843). Samuel Hahnemann (Father of Homeopathy) was a German physician who earned his Doctor of Medicine degree in 1779. It is a therapeutic system of medicine premised on the principle, "*Similia Similibus Curentur*" (like cures like) and law of minimal dose. It is bases on a method of treatment for curing the patient by medicines that possess the power of producing similar symptoms in a healthy human being simulating the natural disease, which in turn can cure the diseased person.

Homeopathy Evolution in India

Homeopathy history in India is as old as when in 1810 when Dr. John Martin Honigberger (disciple of Dr. Samuel Hahnemann) visited India and treated patients with a homeopathic system of medicine. In his second visit in the year 1839, he treated the then ruler of Punjab, Maharaja Ranjit Singh with '*Dulcamara*' for paralysis of vocal cords and edema. Homeopathy was introduced in India in the early 19th century, flourished in Bengal at first, and then spread all over India. Dr. Mahendra Lal Sircar was the first Indian homeopathic physician. The Calcutta Homeopathic Medical College was the first Indian homeopathic medical college established in 1881.

Central Council for Research in Homoeopathy (CCRH)

Central Council for Research in Homoeopathy (CCRH) is an apex research organization under Ministry of AYUSH, Govt. of India. It undertakes, coordinates, develops, disseminates and promotes scientific research in Homoeopathy. The CCRH was formally constituted on 30th March, 1978 as an autonomous organization, registered under the Societies Registration Act XXI, 1860. The CCRH was established to formulate the aims and boost the patterns of research on scientific lines in the Homoeopathy system of medicine in India.

National Commission for Homoeopathy (NCH)

In exercise of the powers conferred by section 18(i) of the 'National Commission for Homeopathy Act, 2020' (15 of 2020), the Central Government has constituted the following Autonomous Boards, namely: Homoeopathy Education Board, Medical Assessment and Rating Board for Homeopathy, and Board of Ethics and Registration for Homeopathy. 'The National Commission for Homeopathy Act, 2020' came into force on 05th July 2021. The aims of NCH is to improve access to quality and affordable medical education in Homeopathy and ensure availability of adequate and high quality Homeopathy medical professionals throughout India.

Definition of 'Homeopathic medicines'

As per Section 2(dd) of the Drugs and Cosmetics Act, '*Homeopathic medicines include any drug which is recorded in Homoeopathic proving or therapeutic efficacy of which has been established through long clinical experience as recorded in authoritative Homeopathic literature of India and abroad and which is prepared according to the techniques of Homeopathic pharmacy and covers combination of ingredients of such Homeopathic medicines but does not include a medicine which is administered by parenteral route*'.

Definition of 'Homeopathy'

As per Section 2(f) of the National Commission for Homeopathy Act, 2020 '*Homeopathy means the Homoeopathic System of Medicine and includes the use of biochemic remedies supplemented by such modern advances, scientific and technological development as the Commission may, in consultation with the Central Government, declare by notification from time to time*'.

Definition of 'Registered Homeopathic Medical Practitioner'

As per the Section 2 (ea) of the Drugs and Cosmetics Act, a "registered Homeopathic medical practitioner" means a person who is registered in the Central Register or a State Register of Homeopathy.

Rules for sale of Homeopathic medicines

Under Part VI(A) of the Drugs and Cosmetics Act, the rules for the sale of homeopathic medicines are prescribed. Following are the rules prescribed under the Drugs Rules for the sale of homeopathic medicines.

1. **Homeopathic Sale License**: As per Rule 67(C) the forms of license to sell, stock or exhibit or offer for sale or distribute Homeopathic medicines by a retail or by wholesale shall be issued in 'Form 20C' or 'Form 20D' as the case may be. Hence, a licensed Homeopathic pharmacy shops, Homeopathic practioners clinics and even Allopathic chemist shops can dispense Homeopathic medicines under the personal supervision of a competent person to deal in Homeopathic medicines. Provided that no license shall be required for exhibiting the Drugs for promotional activities in any fair.

   - Form 20C - Retail Sale Drug License for Homeopathic medicines.
   - Form 20D - Wholesale Drug License for Homeopathic medicines.
   - Form 20C and 20D - Combined Retail and Wholesale License for Homeopathic medicines.
   - Form 20E - Renewal Certificate for Homeopathic Sale License.

   If a Chemist shop already possess a Retail Sale Drug License (RSDL) i.e. Form 20 and 21 then, there is no additional requirement of having a Retail Sale Drug License for homeopathy i.e. Form 20C. However, in case of wholesale, it is mandatory to have a Wholesale Drug License for homeopathy i.e. Form 20D separately, inspite a wholesaler possess a Wholesale Drug License i.e. Form 20B and 21B.

2. **Competent Person for sale of Homeopathic Medicines**: As per the Rule 67(F)(1), conditions to be satisfied before a license in Form 20C or Form 20D is granted for those 'who is in the opinion

of the Licensing Authority competent to deal in Homeopathic medicines' which includes the following qualifications:
(a) Degree in Homeopathy; or
(b) Degree in Pharmacy (B.Pharm); or
(c) Graduation with one-year experience of dealing in Homeopathic medicines in the premises of a registered Homeopathic RMP or a Homeopathy medical store; or
(d) Diploma in Homeopathic Pharmacy; or
(e) Diploma in Homeopathy Medicine and Surgery (DHMS).

3. **Exemption for Homeopathic globules, water or milk sugar**: As per the Rule 67(G)(2) the sale of Homeopathic medicines shall be conducted under the supervision of a person having qualifications referred to in Rule 67(F)(1) and in manufacturer's sealed packing only. However, no competent person is required to dispense Homeopathic medicines in the form of globules, water or milk sugar as per prescription of a Homoeopathic Medical Practitioner.

4. **Exemption under 'Schedule K' for Homeopathic Medicines:** Homeopathic medicines are exempted from the provisions of Chapter IV of the Drugs and Cosmetics Act. It means for sale of Homeopathic medicines there is no requirement of a Homeopathic Registered Medical Practitioner (RMP)'s prescription but, the sale licenses namely: Form 20C (for retail sale) and Form 20D (for wholesale) are mandatorily required.

    o **Schedule K - Serial Number 31:** *Homeopathic Medicines.*
    o **Schedule K - Serial Number 35:** *Homeopathic hair oils having active ingredients up to 3X potency only.*

Class of Drugs	Extent and Conditions of Exemptions
31. Homeopathic medicines	The provisions of Chapter IV of the Act and the rules made thereunder which relates to sale license in Form 20C, subject to the following conditions: - (i) These medicines shall be sold in the original sealed small quantity packings of the licensed

	manufacturers; (ii) Medicines shall be stocked and sold by retail dealers of medicines licensed under rule 61; (iii) Medicines shall be stored separately from other allopathic drugs; (iv) Medicines shall be purchased from a manufacturer or a dealer licensed under these rules; and (v) Purchase and sale records of medicines shall be maintained by the dealer for a minimum period of three years."
35. Homeopathic hair oils having active ingredients up to 3X potency only	The provisions of Chapter IV of the Act and the rules made thereunder which require them to be covered with a sale license in Form 20C subject to the condition that such product has been manufactured under a valid manufacturing license and sold in the original sealed packing of the licensed manufacturers.

5. **Exemption of Expiry Date for 'Dilutions' and 'Back Potencies':** Under paragraph 9, relating to Expiry Date 'homeopathic dilutions' and 'back potencies' are being kept separated from the existing provision of not exceeding 60 months (5 years) from the date of manufacture. It means expiry date is not a mandatory labeling requirement for the homeopathic formulations of 'dilutions' and 'back potencies'.

6. **Sale at more than one place:** As per Rule 67(D), if homeopathic medicines are sold, stocked or distributed from more than one place, a separate application shall be made and a separate license shall be obtained in respect of each place.

7. **Duration of homeopathic sale licenses:** As per Rule 67(E), an original license or a renewed licence unless it is sooner suspended or canceled shall be valid for a period of 'five years' on and from the date on which it is granted or renewed. Provided that if the application for renewal of a licence in force is made before its expiry or if the application is made within six month of its expiry, after payment of additional fee, the license shall continue to be in force until orders are passed on the application and the license shall be deemed to have

expired if application for its renewal is not made within six months after its expiry.

8. **Certificate of renewal:** As per Rule 67(EE), the certificate of renewal of a sale licence in Forms 20C and 20D (Homeopathic Sale Drug Licenses) shall be issued in 'Form 20E'.

9. **Prohibition of quantity and alcohol percentage:** As per Rule 106(B), no Homoeopathic medicine containing more than 12% alcohol v/v (Ethyl Alcohol) shall be packed and sold in packing or bottles of more than 30 ml, except that it may be sold to hospitals/dispensaries in packings or bottles of not more than 100 ml. Hence, it means that a homeopathic medicine retailer can only dispense 30 ml per unit containing not more than 12% of ethyl alcohol. However, a hoemapthic medicine wholesaler can sale upto 100 ml per unit containing not more than 12% of ethyl alcohol to a hospitals and dispensaries.

10. **Conditions of license:** As per Rule 67(G) License in Form 20C or 20D shall be subject to the conditions stated therein and to the following further conditions, namely:
(1) The premises where the Homeopathic medicines are stocked for sale or sold are maintained in a clean condition.
(2) The sale of Homeopathic medicines shall be conducted under the supervision of a person, competent to deal in Homeopathic medicines.
(3) The licensee shall permit an Inspector to inspect the premises and furnish such information as he may require for ascertaining whether the provisions of the Act and the Rules made thereunder have been observed.
(4) The licensee in Form 20D shall maintain records of purchase and sale of Homeopathic medicines containing alcohol together with names and addresses of parties to whom sold.
(5) The licensee in Form 20C shall maintain records of purchase and sale of Homeopathic medicines containing alcohol. No records of sale in respect of Homeopathic potentised preparation in containers of 30 ml. or lower capacity and in respect of mother tinctures made up in quantities upto 60 ml. need to be maintained.
(6) The licensee shall maintain an Inspection Book in Form 35 to enable an Inspector to record his impressions and the defects noticed.

11. **Documents requirement for application of a fresh homeopathic drug sale license (Form 20C & Form 20D):**
    1. Application Form No. 19(B).
    2. GRIPS state government challan of Rs. 250 (Licence Fees)
    3. Additional information Form with recent photograph of experienced qualified person in – Charge.
    4. House Rent Bill. (Xerox). House Tax Bill of proposed premises issued by local municipality / Government Tax Receipt issued by B.L.R.O. in case of Panchayat area.
    5. Appointment letter of qualified person in charge. Madhyamik certificate (Xerox) of a qualified person. 5 years experience certificate of qualified person. Date of birth certificate proof of qualified person.
    6. Copy of partnership, in case of partnership firms. Copy of receipt of registration of firms in case of partnership firm.
    7. Memorandum of Article of Association in case of Limited or Private Limited firm. Extract of resolution taken in the Board of Directors meeting regarding business in drug & to appoint authorized signatory.
    8. List of Directors (In case of Limited or Private Limited, Company)
    9. Sketch plan of the proposed premises with actual dimensions, surroundings and signature of proprietor / partners/ directors.
    10. Required area of the proposed business premises – 108 Sq. Ft. (Carpet area). Required ceiling height – min. 8' Ft. The premises shall be brick built, plastered & floor cemented with R.C.C. roofing. The proposed premises should be completely separated with completely separate and identical entrances. No residential common passage will be allowed.
    11. House owner of the proposed premises should sign himself in full in the House rent bill.
    12. Address of the firm in all related papers must be the same as in House Tax Receipt.

CHAPTER 6

Medical Devices and In Vitro Diagnostics (IVDs) Sale Rule

Introduction

Medical devices in day to day life plays a crucial role in the healthcare sector and are an extraordinarily heterogeneous class of products. The term 'Medical Device' includes such technologically simple items as ice bags and tongue depressors on one end of the continuum and very sophisticated items such as cardiac pacemakers, PET scan, MRI scan and proton therapy devices on the other end. Broadly based on the function of medical devices they may be classified as 'preventive care device', 'assistive care device', 'diagnostic device' and 'therapeutic device'.

- Preventive care medical devices: Blood pressure monitors, Glucometers, Thermometers etc.
- Assistive care medical devices: Wheel chair, Hearing aid etc.
- Diagnostic medical devices: X ray machine, CT Scan machine, Ultrasound machine, Covid 19 test kit, HIV test kit, Blood glucose monitoring system, Blood pressure monitor etc.
- Therpaeutic medical devices: Bed/Chair electric massager, Nebulizer etc.

Background

Medical Devices Rules (MDR), 2017 were notified by the Government vide notification no. GSR 78 (E) dated 31.01.2017 which has been enforced w.e.f. 01.01.2018. The first definition of 'Medical Devices' was introduced in Drugs & Cosmetics Act, 1940 under Section 3(b)(iv) in 1982. Prior to it, there was no definition of Medical Devices. Later, 'In-Vitro Diagnostics' (IVDs) devices for HIV, HbsAg & HCV were notified w.e.f. 01.09.2002 as 'Drug' under section 3(b)(i) of the Drugs and Cosmetics Act. The Medical Devices Rules contains 12 Chapters, 8 Schedules, 97 Rules and 43 Forms.

Regulation of Medical devices in India

1. <u>Central Licensing Authority</u> - The Drugs Controller General of India (DCGI) is the Central Licensing Authority, competent for the enforcement of these rules in matters relating to:
   - Import of all Classes of medical devices;
   - Manufacture of Class C and Class D medical devices;
   - Clinical investigation and approval of investigational medical devices;
   - Clinical performance evaluation and approval of new in vitro diagnostic medical devices and;
   - Coordination with the State Licensing Authorities.

2. <u>State Licensing Authority</u> - The State Drugs Controller, by whatever name called, shall be the State Licensing Authority and shall be the competent authority for enforcement of these rules in matters relating to:
   - Manufacture for sale or distribution of Class A or Class B medical devices;
   - Sale, stock, exhibit or offer for sale or distribution of medical devices of all classes.

Definition of Medical Devices

All devices including an instrument, apparatus, appliance, implant, material or other article, whether used alone or in combination, including a software or an accessory, intended by its manufacturer to be used specially for human beings or animals which does not achieve the primary intended action in or on human body or animals by any pharmacological or immunological or metabolic means, but which may assist in its intended function by such means for one or more of the specific purposes of:

(a) Diagnosis, prevention, monitoring, treatment or alleviation of any disease or disorder

(b) Diagnosis, monitoring, treatment, alleviation or assistance for, any injury or disability

(c) Investigation, replacement or modification or support of the anatomy or of a physiological process

(d) Supporting or sustaining life

(e) Disinfection of medical devices and

(f) Control of conception.

NOTE: For the purpose of these rules, substances used for in vitro diagnosis shall be referred to as in vitro diagnostic medical devices.

Definition of IVDs (In Vitro Diagnostics)

IVDs are substances intended to be used outside human or animal bodies for the diagnosis of any disease or disorder in human beings or animals covered under sub clause (i) of clause (b) of Section 3 of the Drugs and Cosmetics Act, 1940 and IVDs that are notified, from time to time, as a device under sub-clause (iv) of clause (b) of Section 3 of the Drugs and Cosmetics Act, 1940.

Classification of Medical Devices (based on risk assessment)

Based on the risk classification Medical devices and In-Vitro Diagnostics (IVDs) has been classified as:

- Low risk - Class A
- Low moderate risk - Class B
- Moderate high risk - Class C
- High risk - Class D

Exemption for Class A non-measuring & non-sterile medical devices

As per GSR 777 (E) dated 14 Oct, 2022 for 'Class A non-measurable and non-sterile' Medical Devices, no manufacturing or import license will be required, only registration of the product is required on Sugam Portal link (www.cdscomdonline.gov.in). The online registration process will generate a unique 'file number' or 'registration number' which must be included on the product label prior to marketing by the manufacturers or importers.

With this update, the Medical Device (Sixth Amendment) Rules, 2022 exempts Class A non-sterile and non-measuring medical devices from the licensing regime by adding a new Chapter III(B) to the MDR, 2017. Common Class A non-measuring and non-sterile devices include items such as: Scalpels, Gauze, Bandages, Some examination gloves, etc.

NOTE: However, 'Class A sterile and measuring medical devices' will require an import and manufacturer license and these categories of medical devices are not exempted from the licensing regime.

Notified and Non Notified Medical Devices and IVDs

- Notified Medical Devices: Before Medical Devices (Amendment) Rules, 2020 (w.e.f. 01 April, 2020) all 37 Medical Devices and 1 Disinfectant & Insecticides specified in MDR, 2017 are called as 'Notified Medical Devices'.

SN	NOTIFIED MEDICAL DEVICES	NOTIFICATION NO.	NOTIFICATION DATE
1	Disposable Hypodermic Syringes	GSR 365(E)	17 Mar 1989
2	Disposable Hypodermic Needles	GSR 365(E)	17 Mar 1989
3	Disposable Perfusion Sets	GSR 365(E)	17 Mar 1989
4	IVD Devices for HIV, HBsAg, HCV	GSR 601(E)	27 Aug 2002
5	Cardiac Stents	S.O. 1468(E)	06 Oct 2005
6	Drug Eluting Stents	S.O. 1468(E)	06 Oct 2005
7	Catheters	S.O. 1468(E)	06 Oct 2005
8	Intraocular Lenses	S.O. 1468(E)	06 Oct 2005
9	I.V. Cannulae	S.O. 1468(E)	06 Oct 2005
10	Bone Cements	S.O. 1468(E)	06 Oct 2005
11	Heart Valves	S.O. 1468(E)	06 Oct 2005
12	Scalp Vein Set	S.O. 1468(E)	06 Oct 2005
13	Blood Grouping Sera	NA	NA
14	Ligatures, Sutures and Staplers	NA	NA
15	IntraUterine Devices (CuT)	NA	NA
16	Condoms	NA	NA

17	Tubal Rings	NA	NA
18	Surgical Dressings	NA	NA
19	Umbilical tapes	NA	NA
20	Blood/Blood Component Bags	NA	NA
21	Disinfectant & Insecticides specified in MDR, 2017	NA	NA
22	Blood Pressure Monitors	S.O. 5980	01 Jan 2021
23	Digital Thermometers	S.O. 5980	01 Jan 2021
24	Glucometers	S.O. 5980	01 Jan 2021
25	Nebulizers	S.O. 5980	01 Jan 2021
26	X-Ray Machines	GSR 775(E)	08 Feb 2019
27	CT Scan Equipment	GSR 775(E)	08 Feb 2019
28	MRI Equipment	GSR 775(E)	08 Feb 2019
29	PET Equipment	GSR 775(E)	08 Feb 2019
30	Defibrillators	GSR 775(E)	08 Feb 2019
31	Dialysis Machines	GSR 775(E)	08 Feb 2019
32	Bone Marrow Cell Separators	GSR 775(E)	08 Feb 2019
33	All Implantable Medical Devices	GSR 775(E)	08 Feb 2019
34	Ultrasound Devices	NA	NA
35	Ablation Devices	NA	NA
36	Organ Preservation Solution	S.O. 1500(E)	02 Apr 2019
37	Internal Prosthetic Replacements	NA	NA
38	Orthopedic Implants	NA	NA

- Newly Notified Medical Devices: All medical devices except 'notified medical devices' are categorized under the 'Newly Notified Medical Devices' which comprises 24 'Medical Devices' and 3 'In-Vitro Diagnostics' (IVDs)'. Medical devices submitted under the new voluntary rules are referred to as "Non-Regulated Medical Devices".

The registration process will generate a unique 'file number' or 'registration number' on the same day which shall be included on the product label prior to marketing. All class A and B non-regulated medical devices will have to obtain compulsory registration number before Oct, 2022. On the other hand, all class C and D non-regulated medical devices will have to obtain registration number before Oct, 2023.

The 27 categories of 'newly notified medical devices' includes:
1. Anaesthesiology
2. Pain Management
3. Cardiovascular
4. Dental
5. Ear, Nose, Throat (ENT)
6. Gastroenterological
7. Urological
8. General Hospital
9. Operation Theater
10. Respiratory
11. Neurological
12. Personnel use
13. Obstetrical and Gynaecological (OG)
14. Ophthalmic
15. Rehabilitation
16. Physical support
17. Interventional and Radiology
18. Rheumatology
19. Dermatology and Plastic Surgery
20. Pediatric and Neonatology Medical
21. Oncology
22. Radiotherapy
23. Nephrology and Renal care
24. Software
25. IVD Analyser
26. IVD Instrument
27. IVD Software

IVDs (In Vitro Diagnostics) Classification Lists

The Central Drugs Standard Control Organisation (CDSCO) of India has issued a file no. IVD/Misc/196/2020 on 25 Oct 2023 updating several in-vitro diagnostic (IVD) categories and classifications. The updates to IVD classification list include intended use, associated risk, additional IVD categories, and other parameters. The notice advised that the CDSCO has updated two lists under the Medical Device Rules, 2017:

- Annexure A - IVD analyzers – 72 total medical devices (updated and revised).
- Annexure B - IVD instruments – 29 medical devices (updated and revised).
- Annexure C - IVDs Software.
- Annexure D - IVD Specimen Receptacles (added).
- Annexure E - Covid 19, DNA, and mRNA Extraction Kits, etc. (added).

NOTE: *There were no changes made to Annexure C which covers IVD software, although any software that drives a device or influences its use falls in the same class automatically.*

Product standard for Medical Devices

As per Rule 7 under the Chapter II (Regulation of Medical Devices) of the Medical Devices Rules, 2017 a medical device shall have the following standard norms:

1. The medical device shall conform to the standards laid down by the 'Bureau of Indian Standards' established under section 3 of the Bureau of Indian Standards Act, 1985 (63 of 1985) or as may be notified by the Ministry of Health and Family Welfare in the Central Government, from time to time.
2. Where no relevant Standard of any medical device has been laid down under sub-rule (1), such device shall conform to the standard laid down by the 'International Organisation for Standardisation (ISO)' or the 'International ElectroTechnical Commission (IEC)', or by any other 'pharmacopoeial standards'.
3. In case of the standards which have not been specified under sub-rule (1) and sub-rule (2), the device shall conform to the validated manufacturer's standards.

Hence, a manufacturer shall have any one approval of the product standards as per the Rule 7 of the Medical Devices Rules, 2017:

1. Bureau of Indian Standards (BIS), or

2. International Organisation for Standardisation (ISO), or
3. International Electro Technical Commission (IEC), or
4. Any Pharmacopoeial standards, or
5. Any validated manufacturer's standard.

Legal Metrology Rules, 2011

Medical Devices are not exempted under the Legal Metrology Rules. As per Rule 26(C) of Legal Metrology (Packaged Commodities) Rules, 2011 Medical Devices package shall bear mandatory information including:

- Retail Sales Price (in the form of MRP)
- Unit Sale Price
- Country of Origin
- Size and Dimensions of the Commodity
- Consumer Care details

Drug Price Control Order (DPCO), 2013

The NPPA vide Notification dated 31 Mar, 2020 in pursuance of Notification No. SO 648(E), dated 11 Feb, 2020, stated that all medical devices shall be governed under the provisions of the DPCO, 2013 w.e.f. 1st Apr 2020. NPPA also monitors prices of notified medical devices under compulsory licensing framework under Para 20 of the DPCO, 2013 to ensure their MRP is not increased more than 10% in preceding twelve months. Few medical devices prices has been fixed by the NPPA under Para 19 of the DPCO, 2013 includes:

- Coronary Stents
- Knee Implants
- Cardiac Stents
- Drug Eluting Stents
- Condoms
- IntraUterine Devices (Cu-T)
- Oxygen Concentrators
- Pulse Oximeter
- Blood Pressure Monitoring Machine
- Nebulizer
- Digital Thermometer

- Glucometer
- Disposable Hypodermic Syringes
- Disposable Hypodermic Needles
- Disposable Perfusion Sets
- IVD devices of HIV, HBsAg and HCV
- Catheters
- Intraocular Lenses
- I.V. Cannulae
- Bone Cements
- Heart Valves
- Scalp Vein Set
- Orthopedic Implants
- Internal Prosthetic Replacements
- Ablation Devices
- Organ Preservative Solution
- Blood Grouping Sera
- Ligatures, Sutures and Staplers
- Tubal Rings
- Surgical Dressings
- Umbilical tapes
- Blood/Blood Component Bags

Labeling of Medical Devices

As per Rule 44 under Chapter VI of the MDR, 2017 the label of the medical device should bear the following particulars shall be printed in indelible ink on the label, on the shelf pack of the medical device or on the outer cover of the medical device and on every outer covering in which the medical device is packed, namely:

(a) name of the medical device;
(b) details necessary for the user to identify the device and its use;
(c) name of manufacturer and address of manufacturing premises;
(d) net quantity in terms of weight, measure, volume, number of units, as the case may be, and the number of the devices contained in the package expressed in metric system;

(e) month and year of manufacture and expiry (alternately the label shall bear the shelf life of the product) e.g. in case of medical equipment or instruments or apparatus, the date of expiry may not be necessary. The month and the date of expiry shall be preceded by the words "Expiry date" or "Shelf Life;
(f) indication that the device contains medicinal or biological substance;
(g) batch number or lot number preceded by the word "Lot No." or "Lot" or "Batch No." or "B. No.";
(h) to indicate, wherever required, any special storage or handling conditions applicable to the device;
(i) to indicate, if the device is supplied as a sterile product, its sterile state and the sterilization method;
(j) to give, if considered relevant, warnings or precautions to draw the attention of the user of medical device;
(k) to label the device appropriately, if the device is intended for single use;
(l) to overprint on the label of the device, the words "Physician's Sample—Not to be sold", if a medical device is intended for distribution to the medical professional as a free sample;
(m) to provide, except for imported devices, the manufacturing license number by preceding the words "Manufacturing Licence Number" or "Mfg. Lic. No." or "M. L";
(n) to provide on the label, in case of imported devices, by way of stickering, where such details are not already printed, the import license number, name and address of the importer, address of the actual manufacturing premises and the date of manufacture: Provided that the label may bear symbols recognised by the Bureau of Indian Standards or International Organisation for Standardisation (ISO) in lieu of the text and the device safety is not compromised by a lack of understanding on the part of the user, in case the meaning of the symbol is not obvious to the device user;
(o) in case of small sized medical devices on which information cannot be printed legibly, shall include the information necessary for product identification and safety such as information covered by clauses (a), (b), (c), (d), (e), (g), (k), and (m) shall be included.

Repacking of Medical Devices

There is no provision for repacking of Medical Devices in MDR, 2017.

Exemptions of Medical Devices under Eighth Schedule (Rule 90)

Following categories of medical devices are exempted from the provisions of the Medical Devices Rules with certain conditions -

1. Custom made device.
2. Medicated dressings and bandages for first aid.
3. Medical Device supplied to his patient, or any medical device supplied by a Doctor at the request of another such Doctor.
4. Medical devices supplied by a hospital or dispensary maintained or supported by Government or local body
5. Mechanical contraceptives (Condoms, Male condom, Vaginal ring, Copper IUD,
6. Import of small quantity of medical devices donated to a charitable hospital for treatment of patients free of cost by that hospital.

Sale Rule for Medical Devices in India

The Ministry of Health and Family Welfare, Government of India has published the 5th Amendment of Medical Device Rule via General Statutory Rule (G.S.R.) 754(E) on 30th September 2022. This Rule has made provision for Registration Certificate to sell, stock, exhibit, or offer for sale or distribute a medical device including In-Vitro diagnostic device. It means a retailer, wholesaler, or stockist of medical devices including IVDs not having a retail or wholesale drug license (Form 20, 21, 20B, and 21B) must get a Medical device registration certificate (Form MD 42) from the state licensing authority. This Form MD 42 is mandatory from 30 September 2022 for all medical device sellers.

1. **Medical Device Registartion Certificate (Form MD 42):** This medical devices registration certification i.e. Form MD 42 runs parallel to the current requirement of having drug sale licenses (i.e. Form 20 & 21 or Form 20B & 21B) for drugs. The State Licensing Authority (SLA) will be responsible for issuing, approving or rejecting the application made in Form MD 41 (i.e. Application for grant of registration certificate to sell, stock, exhibit or offer for sale or distribute a medical device including in-vitro diagnostic medical device). The State Licensing Authority (SLA) after satisfactory review, will grant the Form MD 42 (i.e. Registration Certificate to sell, stock, exhibit or offer for sale or distribute a medical device including in vitro diagnostic medical device).

Note: If a retailer/wholesaler/distributor has already a valid drug sale license (Form 20 & 21) or (Form 20B & 21B) then there is no requirement to obtain Form MD 42 for sale, stock and distribution of medical devices.

2. **Pre-Licensing requirements for obtaining Form MD 42:** Any individual or entity who intends to sell, stock, exhibit, offer for sale or distribute a medical device, including in-vitro diagnostic medical devices must obtain the medical device registration certificate i.e. Form MD 42 under the Medical Devices Rules. The process for obtaining the certificate is as follows:
   a. Application for a Registration Certificate must be made in Form MD 41 to the State Licensing Authority (SLA).
   b. Fees of Rs. 3000 has to be submitted along with relevant documents, and if found satisfactory after review the authority will grant the Medical Device Registration Certificate in Form MD 42.
   c. Form MD 42 will remain valid in perpetuity as long as a retention fee of Rs. 3000 rupees is paid every 5 years.
   d. The application made under sub-rule (2) shall be accompanied with:
   (i) Fees (Rs. 3000) specified in Second Schedule;
   (ii) Self certificate of compliance with respect to Good Distribution Compliance;
   (iii) Details of the applicant or firm including its constitution, along with identification proof, such as, Aadhar card or PAN card;
   (iv) Documentary evidence in respect of ownership or occupancy on rental of the premises;
   (v) Details of competent technical staff (CTS), under whose direction and supervision the sales activity of medical device shall be undertaken, who shall possess the following educational qualification and experience, namely:
   - *Graduate in any stream from a recognized university; or*
   - *Registered Pharmacist (RP); or*
   - *Intermediate (XII) pass with one-year experience in sale of medical devices;*

   (vi) Brief description on other activities carried out by applicant, namely, storage of drugs, medical items, food products,

stationeries, etc., or any other activities carried out by the applicant in the said premises; and

(vii) An undertaking to the effect that the storage requirements to sell, stock, exhibit or offer for sale or distribute a medical device will be complied with.

3. **Post-licensing requirement for a Form MD 42 registration holder (Rule 87B):**
   - The registration certificate granted under rule 87A shall be displayed at a prominent place in the premises visible to the public.
   - The registration certificate holder shall provide adequate space and proper storage condition for storage of the medical devices.
   - The registration certificate holder shall maintain requisite temperature and lighting as per requirements of such medical devices.
   - The medical devices shall be purchased only from importer or licensed manufacturer or registered/licensed entity.
   - Separate records, in the form of invoice or register or electronic details including software of purchases and sales of medical devices must be retained. These records must show the names and quantities of such medical devices, names and addresses of the manufacturers or importers, batch number or lot number and expiry date (if applicable) shall be maintained.
   - All registers and records referred to in sub-rule (5) shall be open to inspection by a Medical Device Officer who may, if necessary, make enquiries about purchases and sale of the medical devices and may also take samples for testing.
   - All registers and records mentioned under these rules, shall be preserved for a period of not less than two years from the last entry, therein.
   - The registration certificate holder shall maintain an inspection book in Form MD-43 to enable the Medical Devices Officer to record his observations and defects noticed.

Important Forms

1. Form MD 41 - [Sub-rule (2) of Rule 87A] APPLICATION FOR GRANT OF REGISTRATION CERTIFICATE TO SELL, STOCK, EXHIBIT OR OFFER FOR SALE OR DISTRIBUTE A MEDICAL DEVICE INCLUDING IN VITRO DIAGNOSTIC MEDICAL DEVICE.

> **"Form MD-41**
>
> *[See sub-rule (2) of rule 87A]*
>
> **APPLICATION FOR GRANT OF REGISTRATION CERTIFICATE TO SELL, STOCK, EXHIBIT OR OFFER FOR SALE OR DISTRIBUTE A MEDICAL DEVICE INCLUDING *IN VITRO* DIAGNOSTIC MEDICAL DEVICE**
>
> 1. Name of applicant:
> 2. Address of the premises to be registered:
> 3. Contact details of applicant including telephone number, mobile number, fax number and email id:
> 4. Nature and constitution of applicant: (*i.e.* proprietorship, partnership including Limited Liability Partnership, private or public company, society, trust, other to be specified)
> 5. Name, qualification and experience of competent person appointed:
> 6. Fee paid on _____ Rs _____ receipt/challan/transaction Id _____ .
> 7. I have enclosed the documents as specified in the sub-rule (3) of rule 87A of the Medical Devices Rules, 2017.
>
> Place: _____
> Date: _____
>
> Name, designation & signature of
> Director/Proprietor/Partner

1. Form MD 42 - [Sub-rule (4) of Rule 87A and Sub-Rule (1) of Rule 87C] REGISTRATION CERTIFICATE TO SELL, STOCK, EXHIBIT OR OFFER FOR SALE OR DISTRIBUTE A MEDICAL DEVICE INCLUDING IN VITRO DIAGNOSTIC MEDICAL DEVICE.

> **Form MD-42**
>
> *[See sub-rule(4) of rule 87A and sub-rule (1) of rule 87C]*
>
> **REGISTRATION CERTIFICATE TO SELL, STOCK, EXHIBIT OR OFFER FOR SALE OR DISTRIBUTE A MEDICAL DEVICE INCLUDING *IN VITRO* DIAGNOSTIC MEDICAL DEVICE**
>
> Registration No.: _____
>
> 1. M/s, ...(Name of the firm) situated at ....(full address with telephone and e-mail) has been registered to sell, stock, exhibit or offer for sale or distribute a medical device including *in vitro* diagnostic medical device under the Medical Devices Rules, 2017.
>
> 2. Name and qualification of competent person:
>
> 3. This registration is subject to the conditions as specified in the Drugs and Cosmetics Act, 1940 (23 of 1940) and the Medical Devices Rules, 2017.
>
> Place: _____
> Date: _____
>
> State Licensing Authority

2. <u>Form MD 43</u> - [Sub-Rule (8) of Rule 87B] FORM IN WHICH THE INSPECTION BOOK SHALL BE MAINTAINED.

Form MD-43

[*See sub-rule (8) of rule 87B*]

Form in which the Inspection Book shall be maintained

(A) The cover of the inspection book shall contain the following particulars, namely:—

1. The name and address of the registration certificate holder _____

2. Registration certificate number _____

(B) (i) The pages of the inspection book shall be serially numbered and duly stamped by the State Licensing Authority*. The pages, other than the first and the last pages, shall have the following particulars:—

Name and designation of the Medical Device Officer who inspected the premises:

Date of inspection _____

Observations of the Medical Device Officer _____

Signature of the Medical Device Officer

Commonly used Medical Devices including IVDs which requires Form MD 42 for sale, stock and distribution:

SN	Medical Devices	IVDs
1	Blood pressure monitor	Covid-19 test kit
2	Digital thermometer	Pregnancy detection kit
3	Pulse oximeter	Fertility detection kit
4	Medical synringe and needles	HIV detection kit
5	Nebulizer	Blood grouping detection test kit
6	Wheel chair	Blood glucose monitoring system (Glucometer device, Glucometer strips)
7	Contact lens (including coloured lens)	
8	Public mask respirator (2 and 3 ply mask)	
9	Bed/chair electric massager	

10	Mechanical or Powered treadmill	
11	Visual eye testing (Snellen chart)	
12	Ice bag and collar (for pain relief)	
13	Acupuncture kit (for pain relief)	

CHAPTER 7

Registered Medical Practitioner (RMP) and Medicine Prescribing

Introduction

In India, Registered Medical Practitioners (RMP) includes Allopathic Doctor, Dentist, Homeopathic Doctor, Ayurvedic Vaidhya, Siddha Doctor, Unani Doctor, Sowa Rigpa Practitioner and Veterinary Doctor who possess a valid qualification/degree approved by Central or State Government and his/her name for time being is entered in the National or State Medical Register. This registration shall be renewed from time to time as defined under the prescribed under the National Medical Commision Act and Rules thereunder.

Registration of Medical Practitioners and Licence to Practice Medicine Regulations, 2023

1. Any person who obtains a primary medical qualification recognized under the National Medical Commission Act, 2019 and qualifies the National Exit Test held under section 15 of the Act, shall be entitled for grant of registration in NMR (National Medical Register).
2. The Ethics and Medical Registration Board (EMRB) shall maintain a National Register of medical practitioners. The National Register shall contain all the entries of the registered medical practitioners of all State Register maintained by the State Medical Councils.
3. The certificate of license shall contain a registration number which shall be formed in such a way that a Unique Identification Number shall be suffixed with a Code of the concerned State/Union Territory. On approval of the application by the State Medical Council, the same shall be reflected in the National Medical Register and also in the State Medical Register.

4. The licence to practice medicine issued to a registered medical practitioner shall be valid for a period of 5 years after which the medical practitioner shall have to renew the licencing by making an application to the State Medical Council.
5. If any medical practitioner registered with the State Medical Council, desirous to practice medicine in another State may apply to the concerned State through the web portal of the Ethics & Medical Registration Board. On submission of an application for transfer of Licence to Practice, an intimation shall be received by the State Medical Council where the medical practitioner is registered for practice and the State Medical Council within a period of 30 days shall approve the application for transfer of Licence to Practice, if it has no objection thereon.

Definition of Registered Medical Practitioner

1. <u>As per Section 2(ee) of the Drugs Rules</u>, 1945 a "Registered medical practitioner" means a person -
(i) Holding a qualification granted by an authority specified or notified under section 3 of the Indian Medical Degrees Act, 1916 (7 of 1916), or specified in the Schedules to the Indian Medical Council Act, 1956 (102 of 1956); or
(ii) Registered or eligible for registration in a medical register of a State meant for the registration of persons practicing the modern scientific system of medicine [excluding the Homeopathic system of medicine]; or
(iii) Registered in a medical register [other than a register for the registration of Homeopathic practitioners] of a State, who although not falling within sub-clause (i) or sub-clause (ii) is declared by a general or special order made by the State Government in this behalf as a person practicing the modern scientific system of medicine for the purposes of this Act; or
(iv) Registered or eligible for registration in the register of dentists for a State under the Dentists Act, 1948 (16 of 1948); or
(v) Who is engaged in the practice of veterinary medicine and who possesses qualifications approved by the State Government.

Types of valid qualifications of RMP in India (based on medicine system)

1. Allopathy - MBBS, DNB, MD/MS, DM/MCh.
2. Homeopathy - BHMS, MD/MS in Homeopathy.
3. Ayurveda - BAMS, MD/MS in Ayurveda.
4. Siddha - BSMS, MD/MS in Siddha.
5. Unani - BUMS, MD/MS in Unani.
6. Sowa Rigpa - BSRMS, PG in Sowa Rigpa.
7. Dental - BDS/MDS.
8. Veterinary - BVSC/MVSC.

1. **Registered Allopathic Medical Practitioner**: MBBS (Bachelor of Medicine and Bachelor of Surgery) is an undergraduate 5½ years course recognized by the National Medical Commission (NMC) which is in charge of regulating the medical professionals of Allopathic or Western System of Medicine in India, along with registration of Allopathic Doctors who can legally practice in India. MBBS doctors can prescribe only allopathic medicines to the patient. All prescription drugs namely Schedule H, H1, G, X and others which has prescription label warning on its label requires a valid allopathic RMP's prescription for sale of allopathic prescription drugs. MD/MS/DNB are the post graduation courses which can be done after completing MBBS. Besides this DM/MCh can also be done after completing MD/MS/DNB in allopathy.

2. **Registered Homeopathic Medical Practitioner:** BHMS (Bachelor of Homeopathic Medicine and Surgery) is an undergraduate 5½ years course recognized by the National Commission for Homeopathy (NCH) which controls and manage the medical education of Homoeopathy courses in India. MD/MS is the post graduation course which can be done after completing BHMS. Besides this PhD in homeopathy can also be done after completing MD/MS in homeopathy. A registered homeopathic medical practitioner can prescribe only homeopathic medicines to the patient.

3. **Registered Ayurvedic Medical Practitioner:** BAMS (Bachelor of ayurvedic medicine and surgery) is an undergraduate 5½ years course recognized by the National Commission For Indian System Of Medicine (NCISM) which is in charge of regulating the medical professionals of Indian System of Medicine in India, along with registration of Ayurvedic Doctors who can legally practice in India.

BAMS doctors can prescribe only ayurvedic medicines to the patient. Besides this, ayurvedic drugs which falls under the category of Schedule E1 drugs requires a valid ayurvedic RMP's prescription for sale due to its poisonous and toxic nature. MD/MS is the post graduation course which can be done after completing BAMS. Besides this PhD in ayurveda can also be done after completing MD/MS in ayurveda.

4. **Registered Siddha Medical Practitioner:** BSMS (Bachelor of siddha medicine and surgery) is an undergraduate 5½ years course recognized by the National Commission For Indian System Of Medicine (NCISM) which is in charge of regulating the medical professionals of Indian System of Medicine in India, along with registration of Siddha Doctors who can legally practice in India. BSMS doctors can prescribe only siddha medicines to the patient. Besides this, siddha drugs which falls under the category of Schedule E1 drugs requires a valid siddha RMP's prescription for sale due to its poisonous and toxic nature. MD/MS is the post graduation course which can be done after completing BSMS. Besides this PhD in siddha can also be done after completing MD/MS in siddha.

5. **Registered Unani Medical Practitioner:** BUMS (Bachelor of unani medicine and surgery) is an undergraduate 5½ years course recognized by the National Commission For Indian System Of Medicine (NCISM) which is in charge of regulating the medical professionals of Indian System of Medicine in India, along with registration of Unani Doctors who can legally practice in India. BUMS doctors can prescribe only unani medicines to the patient. Besides this, unani drugs which falls under the category of Schedule E1 drugs requires a valid unani RMP's prescription for sale due to its poisonous and toxic nature. MD/MS is the post graduation course which can be done after completing BUMS. Besides this PhD in unani can also be done after completing MD/MS in unani.

6. **Registered Sowa Rigpa Medical Practitioner:** 'MenpaKachupa' or BSRMS (Bachelor of Sowa-Rigpa Medicine and Surgery) is an undergraduate 5½ years course recognized by the National Commission For Indian System Of Medicine (NCISM) which is in charge of regulating the medical professionals of Indian System of Medicine in India, along with registration of Sowa Rigpa Doctors who can legally practice in India. PG in sowa rigpa or

'MenrempaChugwa' is the post graduation course which can be done after completing BSRMS.

7. **Registered Dental Practitioner:** BDS (Bachelor of Dental Surgery) is an undergraduate 5 years course recognized by the Dental Council of India (DCI) which is in charge of regulating the dental professionals along with registration of dentists who can legally practice in India. Dentistry comes under allopathy only hence, a registered dental practitioner can prescribe few allopathic prescription drugs related to the teeth or mouth/oral/teeth conditions which includes but not limited to certain analgesics (pain killers), certain antibiotics, multivitamins, and Gastrointestinal drugs like for GERD (gastro esophegal reflux disorder) or hyperacidity. Obviously a Dentist will not prescribe drugs for things which aren't related with teeth or mouth conditions. Example a dentist cannot prescribe allopathic drugs for metabolic disorders (like diabetes), antipsychotic drugs, obstetrics and gynecological related issues. MDS is the post graduation courses which can be done after completing BDS. Besides this PhD in dentistry can also be done after completing MDS in dentistry.

8. **Registered Veterinary Practitioner:** BVSc & AH (Bachelor of Veterinary Science and Animal Husbandry) is an undergraduate 5½ years course recognized by the Veterinary Council of India (VCI) which is in charge of regulating the veterinary medical professionals along with registration of veterinary doctors who can legally practice in India. It deals with the study of medical diagnostics, and treatment of diseases of the animals. After BVSc & AH, students can also apply for post graduation degrees like MVSC & AH (Master of Veterinary Science and Animal Husbandry), or other veterinary related courses.

CHAPTER 8

Registered Pharmacist (RP) and Prescription Drugs Dispensing

Definition of Registered Pharmacist

As per Section 2(i) of the Pharmacy Act, 1948 a "registered pharmacist" means a person whose name is for the time being entered in the register of the State in which he is for the time being residing or carrying on his profession or business of pharmacy.

Registration of Pharmacist under State Pharmacy Council

Section 31 of the Pharmacy Act, 1948 (Qualifications for entry on first register) - A person who has attained the age of 18 years shall be entitled on payment of the prescribed fee to have his name entered in the first register if he/she resides, or carries on the business or profession of pharmacy, in the State and:

a. Holds a degree or diploma in pharmacy or pharmaceutical chemistry or a chemist and druggist diploma of an Indian University or a State Government, as the case may be, or a prescribed qualification granted by an authority outside India, OR

b. Holds a degree of an Indian University other than a degree in pharmacy or pharmaceutical chemistry, and has been engaged in the compounding of drugs in a hospital or dispensary or other place in which drugs are regularly dispensed on prescriptions of medical practitioners for a total period of not less than three years, OR

c. Has passed an examination recognised as adequate by the State Government for compounders or dispensers, OR

d. Has been engaged in the compounding of drugs in a hospital or dispensary or other place in which drugs are regularly dispensed on prescriptions of medical practitioners for a total period of not less than five years prior to the date notified under Section 30 (2).

Renewal of Pharmacist Registration

Section 34 of the Pharmacy Act, 1948 - Every Registered Pharmacist has to renew his/her registration from respective State Pharmacy Council time to time which differs from state to state. Every State Pharmacy Council has its own prescribed renewal fees and the validity.

Section 34 of the Pharmacy Act, 1948:
1. As The State Government may, by notification in the Official Gazette, direct that for the retention of a name on the register after the 31st day of December of the year following the year in which the name is first entered on the register, there shall be paid annually to the State Council such renewal fee as may be prescribed , and where such direction has been made, such renewal fee shall be due to be paid before the first day of April of the year to which it relates.
2. Where a renewal fee is not paid by the due date, the Registrar shall remove the name of the defaulter from the register: Provided that a name so removed may be restored to the register on such conditions as may be prescribed.
3. On payment of the renewal fee, the Registrar shall issue a receipt therefor and such receipt shall be proof of renewal of registration.

Duties of Registered Pharmacist (applicable for retail sale only)

1. <u>Pre-dispensation Prescription validation</u> - Before drug dispensation an endorsed Registered Pharmacist shall validate the prescription for:
   (a) Patient's name and address,
   (b) Medicine name, quantity, dose, and frequency,
   (c) Date of appointment,
   (d) Doctor's name, address, qualification, registration number and his/her signature with date.

Once the Prescription is dispensed, it is the duty of the endorsed registered pharmacist to mention the name and address of the pharmacy with date of medicine dispensation to the patient to avoid misuse of the prescription with 'n' number of times.

Drugs	Contains	Drugs Rules	Interpretation

Rules			
Drugs Rule 65(9)	Dispensing Requirements	(a) Substances specified in Schedule H and Schedule H1 or Schedule X shall not be sold by retail except on and in accordance with the prescription of a Registered Medical Practitioner and in the case of substances specified in Schedule X, the prescriptions shall be in duplicate, one copy of which shall be retained by the licensee for a period of two years. (b) The supply of drugs specified in Schedule H and Schedule H1 or Schedule X to Registered Medical Practitioners, Hospitals, Dispensaries and Nursing Homes shall be made only against the signed order in writing which shall be preserved by the licensee for a period of two years.	(a) Any Prescription drugs (Sch. H, H1, X, G or have prescription label caution warning) shall not be sold by a retail without a RMP's valid Prescription to the Patient or Customer. Schedule X drugs prescription shall be preserved for min. 2 years in retail. (b) Any supply of the Prescription drugs (Sch. H, H1, X, G or have prescription label caution warning) to a Doctor, Hospital, Clinic, Dispensary or Nursing Home shall be made only against signed order by the retail endorsed registered pharmacist and this record shall be preserved for min. 2 years.
Drugs Rule 65(10)	Prescription Requirements	For the purposes of clause (9) a prescription shall: (a) Be in writing and be signed by the person giving it with his usual signature and be dated by him.	A prescription shall: • Be in writing • Have Doctor's Signature with date • Have Name and Address of Patient • Have Total Amount/Quantity (1 strip, 1 vial, 1

		(b) Specify the name and address of the person for whose treatment it is given, or the name and address of the owner of the animal if the drug is meant for veterinary use. (c) Indicate the total amount of the medicine to be supplied and the dose to be taken.	bottle etc.) • Have Total Dose (mg, gm, ml etc.)
Drugs Rule 65(11)	Dispensing Rule	The person dispensing a prescription containing a drug specified in Schedule H, Schedule H1 and Schedule X shall comply with the following requirements in addition to other requirement of these rules: (a) The prescription must not be dispensed more than once unless the prescriber has stated thereon that it may be dispensed more than once. (b) If the prescription contains a direction that it may be dispensed a stated number of times or at stated intervals it must not be dispensed otherwise than in accordance with the directions.	

			(c) At the time of dispensing there must be noted on the prescription above the signature of the prescriber, the name and address of the seller and the date on which the prescription is dispensed.	
Drugs Rule 65(11)(A)	Prescription Medicine Substitution		No person dispensing a prescription containing substance specified in Schedule H, H1 and X may supply any other preparation, whether containing the same substance or not, in lieu thereof.	In case on the prescription if only the generic name of the medicine is mentioned (e.g. Metformin 500 mg) then the endorsed registered pharmacist can substitute it with any branded medicines (like Gluformin 500 mg tablet or Melmet 500 mg tablet).

Standard Prescription Format: A Prescription is a written instruction for medicine from a Registered Medical Practitioner (RMP). There is a link between a RMP and pharmacist when it comes to prescribing. Doctors, Pharmacists and Patients are inter connected in this as *Physician (RMP) → Pharmacist → Patient.*

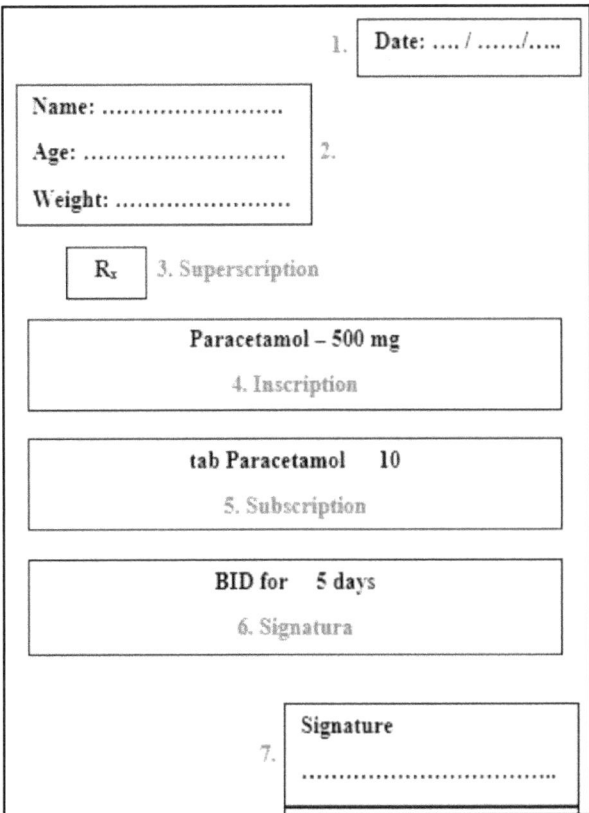

Fig: Parts of a valid Prescription.

The prescription should have following particulars pertaining to Doctor, Patient and Medicines as indicated below:

1. Doctor's full name - Under Drugs Rule 65(3) and it is mandatory to mention name of the doctor as mentioned in her/his registration certificate.
2. Doctor's qualifications - Pharmacist should know that the prescription is valid and to know competency and genuineness of prescriber, the prescription shall bear Doctor's primary qualification such as MBBS/MD/MS/MCh. However, under the Drugs Rules it is not mandatory.
3. Doctor's registration number - Prescription shall bear the registration number of doctor's registration with their respective state medical council. However, under the Drugs Rules it is not mandatory.
4. Doctor's address - Under the Drugs Rules 65(3) it is mandatory to mention the address of the doctor. It is important for the patient and

pharmacist should know where the prescriber/doctor is practicing like address of clinic, hospital or nursing home or own residence. The prescription shall have telephone number (Landline/Mobile) or e-mail ID of the doctor which in turn will help the patient as well as pharmacist to contact doctor, if required.

5. <u>Date of prescription</u> - As per the Drugs Rule 65(10) a prescription shall be dated so that pharmacists should know the validity of prescription to avoid its misuse.
6. <u>Doctor's signature & date</u> - As per the Drugs Rule 65(10) a prescription shall be signed by the person issuing it with her / his usual signature i.e. full signature of prescriber/doctor with date.
7. <u>Doctor's seal/stamp</u> - To avoid misuse of blank or fake prescription and to safeguard patients from quacks and unqualified doctors, the prescription shall have a doctor's seal/stamp with his/her full name, qualifications and registration number below his signature.
8. <u>Prescription serial number</u> - For track and trace a prescriptions' record it must bear a serial number.
9. <u>Patient's full name and address</u> - As per the Drugs Rule 65(10), a valid prescription shall bear the full name and address of the person (i.e. patient) for whose treatment it is given. Patient's Address or contact is essential as pharmacists can get in touch with patients in case of any drug recall or dispensing error.
10. <u>Patient's gender, age and weight</u> - Patient's gender, age and weight are vital factors as drug dosages might vary with age and weight. Gender is important as many drugs are gender specific like gynecological drugs are only for female patient.
11. <u>Complete name of the medicine</u> - Either generic or brand name of the medicine is required on the prescription. E.g. 'Azithral 500 mg tablet' ('Azithral' - brand name, '500 mg' - strength or dose and 'tablet' - dosage form).
12. <u>Dosing instruction</u> - A valid prescription shall bear proper dosing instructions that could be easily understood by patient in any language. E.g. 1 tablet (after breakfast), 1 tablet (after dinner) or 1 tablet (empty stomach) etc.
13. <u>Total quantity and duration (frequency)</u> - A valid prescription shall mention the total quantity of the medicines and duration (frequency) of the treatment. E.g. 'Azithral 500 mg tablet - 1 tablet - bid for 7 days' [total quantity = 14 tablets].

```
                        Doctor's Name
                   Qualification (eg MBBS, MD)
         Regn. No.: .................................................(ALLOPATHY)
              Full Address, Contacts: (telephone No. E-mail etc.)
                                                        Date

Name of the Patient.............................................................

Address*.........................................................................

Age & Sex .............................. weight**

Rx
1)   Name of Medicine***
     Strength, dosage instruction, duration & total quantity***

2)   - do -
3)   - do-
                                                   Doctor's signature
                                                        Stamp
       DISPENSED

Date: ............ Pharmacist: ....................

Name of Pharmacy: .............................
        City
_____

*Postal address/E-mail/Mobile

Number **for Paediatric Patients ***

in capital letters only
_____

Minimum size of the prescription blank should be (a) 14 X 21 cm (A5 size) & (b) XI x XI cm size.
```

Fig: Sample prescription format proposed by the Medical Council of India for registered Doctors.

Duties of a Registered Pharmacist at Pharmacy

A Registered Pharmacist as a custodian of the pharmacy should ensure following good pharmacy practises are followed:

- The entry point of pharmacy should be clearly marked with the word "PHARMACY" or "CHEMISTS AND DRUGGISTS" (whichever is applicable) along with name, address and GST number of licensee as mentioned in the drug sale license in English and local language (like bengali, tamil, punjabi, gujarati etc.)

- Exterior and interiors of the pharmacy should be maintained neat and clean.
- Pharmacy should be free from rodents and pests/insects and pest control measures should be taken from time to time.
- Pharmacy should be equipped with refrigerated storage facilities (validated from time to time) and should be available for drugs like insulin requiring storage at cold temperature. Also there should be constant supply of energy especially for the refrigerator(s).
- Ambient temperature (below 25 degree celsius) in the pharmacy should be maintained within the stipulated range to prevent deterioration of various medicines stored at room temperature conditions.
- Pharmacist should pack cold chain medicine in cold packs only with sufficient ice packs and then hand over it to patient/customer to maintain its uniform temperature between +2 to +8°C till last mile delivery.
- All Registered Pharmacists in the pharmacy should at all times, wear a neat white apron/coat with badge containing details of pharmacist with words 'Registered Pharmacist', 'Name of Pharmacist', and 'Registration number'.
- All necessary statutory documents (e.g. drug sale license, registrations, permissions, etc.) for operating a pharmacy must be adequately maintained and should be displayed at prominent place for public view. Only endorsed Registered Pharmacist Person is authorized to sign all the sales and purchase invoices on behalf of the licensee.
- All operational documents (e.g. purchase invoices, sales invoices, and other statutory documents should be maintained and archived as prescribed under the Drugs Rules and applicable laws.
- Pharmacist shall ensure that all medicines should be purchased from the drug licensed wholesaler only.
- Drugs, which have already expired, should be stored separately in a shelf bearing the label "Expired Goods - Not For Sale".
- Pharmacist should not never substitute branded allopathic prescription medicines until and unless confirmed from the RMP and with patient's consent.

- Pharmacist should maintain a Drug Inspector Inspection booklet (Form 35 for drug sale license) and (Form MD 43 for Medical device sale license/registration) in the premise.
- Pharmacist should always maintain his/her attendance record with date and in/out time.
- Pharmacist should always check prescription for details like Doctor's name/address/registration number, Patient's name/address/age/gender, Medicine name/ strength/ dosage/ quantity supplied, Dosage instruction to patient, Refill information (if any), Date of consultation/ appointment, Doctor's signature with date.
- Pharmacist should always mention the name, address of pharmacy and dispensing date on the prescription above Doctor's signature.
- Pharmacist shall maintain a separate record/register of sale of Schedule H1 medicines at the time of the supply, giving the name and address of the prescriber, the name of the patient, the name of the medicine and the quantity supplied. Such records shall be maintained for three years and be open for inspection.

CHAPTER 9

Part VI - Sale of Drugs other than Homeopathic Medicines

(Drugs Rules Applicable only for Allopathic Medicines)

- Rule 59(1) - The State Government shall appoint Licensing Authorities for the purpose of this Part for such areas as may be specified.

    Interpretation -
    Rule 59(1) - The State Government has power to appoint the officials in the State Licensing Authority (SLA), State Drug Control Department under the Department of Health & Family Welfare of State Governement.

- Rule 59(2) - Applications for the grant or renewal of a license to sell, stock, exhibit or offer for sale or distribute drugs, other than those included in Schedule X, shall be made in Form 19 accompanied by a fee of rupees one thousand and five hundred, or Form 19(A) accompanied by a fee of rupees five hundred, as the case may be, or in the case of drugs included in Schedule X shall be made in Form 19(C) accompanied by a fee of rupees five hundred, to the licensing authority: Provided that in the case of an itinerant vendor or an applicant who desires to establish a shop in a village or town having population of 5,000 or less, the application in Form 19(A) shall be accompanied by a fee of rupees ten.

    Interpretation -
    Rule 59(2) - For the Allopathic Drugs Sale License (Retail and Wholesale) the application has to be made in the 'Form 19' for the Schedule C and C1 except Schedule X Drugs which includes Form 20, 21, 20B, 21B with fees of Rs. 1500 each. Hence, Retail sale drug license (Form 20, 21) total application fees is Rs. 3000 and Wholesale drug

license (Form 20B, 21B) total application fees is Rs. 3000. For the Allopathic Restricted Sale License (Retail) the application has to be made in the 'Form 19(A)' for the Household remedies which includes Form 20A and 21A with fees of total Rs. 500. In case the household remedies shop is located in the place with a population less than 5000 then, total fees for issue of the allopathic restricted drug sale license is Rs. 10 only.

- Rule 59(3) - A fee of rupees one hundred and fifty shall be paid for a duplicate copy of a licence to sell, stock, exhibit or offer for sale or distribute drugs, other than those included in Schedule X, or for a licence to sell, stock, exhibit or offer for sale or distribute drugs, included in Schedule X, if the original is defaced, damaged or lost: Provided that in the case of itinerant vendor or an applicant who desires to establish a shop in a village or town having a population of 5,000 or less, the fee for a duplicate copy of a licence if the original is defaced, damaged or lost, shall be rupees two.

Interpretation -
Rule 59(3) - A fees of Rs. 150 for each Form 20, 21, 20A, 21A, 20B, 21B, 20F, 20G is chargeable if the applicant's license is lost, defaced or damaged and needs a duplicate drug sale license. It means for issue of a duplicate copy of an allopathic retail sale drug license total fees of Rs. 300, allopathic wholesale drug license total fees of Rs. 300 and Schedule X (retail and wholesale) total fees of Rs. 300 will be charged. In the Form 19A (Form 20A, 21A) household remedies shop is located in a place with a population less than 5000 then, total fees for issue of the duplicate copy restricted drug sale license is Rs. 2 only.

- Rule 59(4) - Application for renewal of a licence to sell, stock, exhibit or offer for sale or distribute drugs, after its expiry but within six months of such expiry shall be accompanied by a fee of rupees one thousand and five hundred plus an additional fee at the rate of rupees five hundred per month or part thereof in Form 19, rupees five hundred plus an additional fee at the rate of rupees two hundred and fifty per month or part thereof in Form 19-A and rupees five hundred plus an additional fee at the rate of rupees two hundred and fifty per month or part thereof in Form 19C: Provided that in the case of an itinerant vendor or an applicant desiring to open a shop in a village or town having a population of 5,000 or less the application for such renewal shall be accompanied by a fee of rupees ten, plus an additional fee at the rate of rupees eight per month or part thereof.

Interpretation -
Rule 59(4) -

Application Form	Drug Sale License	License Type	Fresh	Renewal	Late fees per month (only for 6 months)	Duplicate copy fees
19	Form 20	Retail Allopathy	Rs. 1500	Rs. 1500	Rs. 500	Rs. 150
19	Form 21	Retail Allopathy	Rs. 1500	Rs. 1500	Rs. 500	Rs. 150
19	Form 20B	Wholesale Allopathy	Rs. 1500	Rs. 1500	Rs. 500	Rs. 150
19	Form 21B	Wholesale Allopathy	Rs. 1500	Rs. 1500	Rs. 500	Rs. 150
19A	Form 20A	Retail Restricted	Rs. 500	Rs. 500	Rs. 250	Rs. 150
19A	Form 21A	Retail Restricted	Rs. 500	Rs. 500	Rs. 250	Rs. 150
19A*	Form 20A*	Retail Restricted	Rs. 10	Rs. 10	Rs. 8	Rs. 2
19A*	Form 21A*	Retail Restricted	Rs. 10	Rs. 10	Rs. 8	Rs. 2
19AA	Form 20BB	Motor Vehicle	Rs. 500	Rs. 500	Rs. 250	Rs. 150
19AA	Form 21BB	Motor Vehicle	Rs. 500	Rs. 500	Rs. 250	Rs. 150
19C	Form 20F	Retail - Schedule X	Rs. 500	Rs. 500	Rs. 250	Rs. 150
19C	Form 20G	Wholesale - Schedule X	Rs. 500	Rs. 500	Rs. 250	Rs. 150

In case of itinerant vendors or applicants who desire to establish a shop in a town or village having population 5000 or less.

- Rule 60 - A licensing authority may with the approval of the State Government by an order in writing delegate the power to sign licences and such other powers as may be specified in the order to any other person under his control.
  Interpretation -
  Rule 60 - The State Licensing Authority with approval from the State Governement in the form of written order can delegate power to any other person under his control who can approve and sign all licenses and other powers like inspection etc. which is under his control.

- Rule 61(1) - Forms of licences to sell drugs. (1) a license to sell, stock, exhibit or offer for sale or distribute drugs other than those specified in Schedules C, C(1) and X and by retail on restricted licence or by wholesale, shall be issued in Form 20, Form 20A or Form 20B, as the case may be: Provided that a licence in Form 20A shall be valid for only such drugs as are specified in the licence.
  Interpretation -
  Rule 61(1) - Form of a drug sale license shall be issued by the State Licesing Authority (SLA) for the sale, stock and distribution of the allopathic drugs (except Schedule X drugs) shall be issued as a Allopathic Retail Sale Drug License in Form 20 & 21, Allopathic Wholesale Drug License in Form 20B & 21B, and Allopathic Restricted Sale License (for sale of household remedies) in Form 20A & 21A.

- Rule 61(2) - A licence to sell, stock, exhibit or offer for sale or distribute drugs specified in Schedule C and C(1) excluding those specified in Schedule X, by retail on restricted licence or by wholesale shall be issued in Form 21, Form 21A or Form 21B, as the case may be: Provided that a licence in Form 21A shall not be granted for drugs specified in Schedules C and shall be valid for only such Schedule C(1) drugs as are specified in the license.
  Interpretation -
  Rule 61(2) - For stock, sale and distribution of allopathic drugs (Schedule C and C1 except Schedule X) the drug sale license shall be in the Form 21, 21A and 21B. However, for sale, stock and distribution of allopathic restricted drugs (i.e. household remedies) Form 21A

shall not be granted for Schedule C drugs and shall be applicable for Schedule C1 drugs only.

- Rule 61(3) - A licence to sell, stock, exhibit or offer for sale or distribute drugs specified in Schedule X by retail or by wholesale shall be issued in Form 20F or Form 20G as the case may be.
  Interpretation -
  Rule 61(3) - For stock, sale and distribution of allopathic Schedule X drugs, a drug sale license shall be issued by the State Licensing Authority (SLA) in Form 20F (for retail sale) and in Form 20G (for wholesale).

- Rule 62 - Sale at more than one place. If drugs are sold or stocked for sale at more than one place, separate application shall be made, and a separate license shall be issued, in respect of each such place: Provided that this shall not apply to itinerant vendors who have no specified place of business and who will be licensed to conduct business in a particular area within the jurisdiction of the licensing authority.
  Interpretation -
  Rule 62 -Drug sale licenses (Form 20, 21, 20B, 21B, 20A, 21A, 20C, 20D, 20F and 20G) are always location specific. It means if drugs (allopathic and homeopathic) are sold at more than one location then, separate drug sale license needs to be applied for that particular location. Hence, thumb rule of 'ONE DRUG SALE LICENSE - ONE LOCATION' always prevails. Since, the drug sale license is issued by the State Licensing Authority, an applicant needs to apply for a drug sale license in that particular state under which its jurisdiction falls. For Form 21A (itinerant vendors) this rule shall not apply for location specific but shall be within jurisdiction of that State Licensing Authority only.

- Rule 62(A) - Restricted licences in Forms 20A and 21A.
  (a) Restricted licences in Forms 20A and 21A shall be issued subject to the discretion of the Licensing Authority, to dealers or persons in respect of drugs whose sale does not require the supervision of a qualified person.
  (b) Licences to itinerant vendors shall be issued only in exceptional circumstances for bona fide travelling agents of firms dealing in drugs or for a vendor who purchases drugs from a licensed dealer for

distribution in sparsely populated rural areas where other channels of distribution of drugs are not available.

(c) The licensing authority may issue a license in Form 21A to a travelling agent of a firm but to no other class of itinerant vendors for the specific purpose of distribution to medical practitioners or dealers, samples of biological and other special products specified in Schedule C.

Provided that travelling agents of licensed manufacturers, agents, of such manufacturers and importers of drugs shall be exempted from taking out licence for the free distribution of samples of medicines among members of the medical profession, hospitals, dispensaries and the medical institution or research institutions.

Interpretation -

Rule 62(A) -

(a) Allopathic Restricted Drug sale licenses (Form 20A, 21A) shall be under the purview of the State Licensing Authority which will not require the employment and supervision of a Qualified Persons (Registered Pharmacist or Competent Person).

(b) Drug Sale License for itinerant vendors or a temporary stall holder selling drugs shall be only issued for registered travel agents and firms dealing in drugs or wholesaler purchasing drugs from a licensed delaer for distribution in the rural areas with very few population where drug distribution to the people is a problem.

(c) Allopathic Restricted Drug sale licenses (21A) for the drugs specified in Schedule C1 (except Schedule X drugs) can be issued by a State Licensing Authority to a travel agent of a firm but not to itinerant vendor or a temporary stall holder selling drugs for distribution of drugs to Doctors or Dealers for Schedule C drugs.

Provided that, the registered travel agents and registered agents of the drug manufacturers/importers shall be exempted from the requirement of having a drug sale license for the free drug sample distribution among members of the medical profession, hospitals, dispensaries and the medical institution or research institutions.

- Rule 62(B) - Conditions to be satisfied before a licence in Form 20A or Form 21A is granted.

(1) A licence in Form 20A or Form 21A shall not be granted to any person, unless the authority empowered to grant the licence is satisfied that the premises in respect of which the licence is to be granted are adequate and equipped with proper storage accommodation for

preserving the properties of drugs to which the licence applies: Provided that this condition shall not apply in the case of licence granted to itinerant vendors.

(2) In granting a licence under Rule 62A the authority empowered to grant it shall have regard to:

(i) the number of licences granted in the locality during one year immediately preceding; and

(ii) the occupation, trade or business carried on by such applicant : Provided that the licensing authority may refuse to grant or renew a licence to any applicant or licensee in respect of whom it is satisfied that by reason of his conviction of an offence under the Act or these Rules or the previous cancellation or suspension of any licence granted thereunder, he is not a fit person to whom a licence should be granted under this rule.

(3) Any person who is aggrieved by the order passed by the licensing authority in sub-rule (1) may, within 30 days from the date of the receipt of such order appeal to the State Government and the State Government may, after such enquiry into the matter as it considers necessary and after giving the appellant an opportunity for representing his views in the matter make such order in relation thereto as it thinks fit.

Interpretation -

Rule 62(B)(1) - Allopathic Restricted Drug sale licenses (Form 20A, 21A) shall not be granted by the State Licensing Authority if the applicant do not fulfill the condition of license like proper drug storage accommodation is not there which is required for maintaining the drug properties. However, this condition will be not applicable for the itinerant vendor or a temporary stall holder selling drugs.

Rule 62(B)(2) - Regarding the granting of a drug sale license under the Rule 62A (i.e. Restricted licences in Forms 20A and 21A - Household Remedies items) the State Licensing Authority is empowered to grant regarding - (i) number of drug sale license (Form 20A and 21A) granted in last 1 year immediately preceding (ii) occupation, trade, business carried out by such applicant - Provided that the State Licensing Authority may refuse to grant or renew a licence to any applicant due to the reasons like 'applicant previous conviction of an offence record under the Drugs and Cosmetics Act and Rules thereunder' or 'any previous drug sale license cancellation or suspension' or 'applicant does not qualify for the eligibility for license application' to whom a licence should be granted under this rule.

Rule 62(B)(3) - Any person who is not satisfied by the order passed by the state licensing authority regarding suspension or cancellation or not granting license within 30 days from the date of the receipt of such order can file appeal to the State Government against such order of State licensing authority. The State Government may, after such enquiry into the matter may decide and give the opportunity to the appellant (license applicant) for representing his views in the matter make such order in relation thereto as it thinks fit.

- Rule 62(C) - Application for licence to sell drugs by wholesale or to distribute the same from a motor vehicle.

  (1) - Application for the grant or renewal of a licence to sell by wholesale or to distribute from a motor vehicle shall be made to the Licensing Authority in Form 19AA and shall be accompanied by [a fee of rupees five hundred]: Provided that if the applicant applies for the renewal of a licence after its expiry but within six months of such expiry, the fee payable for renewal of such licence shall be [rupees five hundred plus an additional fee at the rate of rupees two hundred and fifty per month or part thereof].

  (2) - A fee of [rupees one hundred and fifty] shall be paid for a duplicate copy of a licence issued under this rule, if the original is defaced, damaged or lost.

  Interpretation -

  Rule 62(C)(1) - The application form for getting drug sale license from a motor vehicle shall be made in application form no. 19AA with a prescribed fees of Rs. 500. Provided that, applicant applies for the this license renewal after its expiry (whichsoever is 5 years) within time period of 6 months after license expiry date. The fees payable for license renewal shall be Rs. 500 and extra amount of Rs. 250 per month.

  Rule 62(C)(2) - If Form 20BB and 21BB (Motor vehicle drug sale license) is lost, defaced or damaged then the licensee shall pay a prescribed fees of Rs. 150 for issue of duplicate copy of the license.

- Rule (62)(D) - Form of licences to sell drugs by wholesale or distribute drugs from a motor vehicle. A licence shall be issued for sale by wholesale or for distribution from a motor vehicle of drugs other than those specified in Schedule C and Schedule C(1) in Form 20BB and of drugs specified in Schedule C and Schedule C(1) in Form 21BB : Provided that such a licence shall not be required in a case where a public carrier or a hired vehicle is used for transportation or distribution of drug.

Interpretation -

Rule 62(D) - Drug sale license from a motor vehicle shall be issued for sale by wholesale or for distrbiution from a motor vehicle (except Schedule C and C1 in Form 20BB), and (Schedule C and C1 in Form 21BB). Provided that, this motor vehicle drug sale licence (Form 20BB and 21BB) is not required in a case where a 'public carrier transport' or a 'hired vehicle' is used for transportation or distribution of drug.

- Rule 63 - Duration of licence. An original licence or a renewed licence to sell drugs, unless sooner suspended or cancelled, shall be valid for a period of five years on and from the date on which it is granted or renewed : Provided that if the application for renewal of licence in force is made before its expiry or if the application is made within six months of its expiry, after payment of additional fee, the licence shall continue to be in force until orders are passed on the application. The licence shall be deemed to have expired if application for its renewal is not made within six months after its expiry.

  Interpretation -

  Rule 63 - The validity of a drug sale license (Form 20, 21, 20B, 21B, 20A, 21A, 20F, 20G, 20BB, 21BB) shall be 5 years from the date of grant of license until and unless suspended or cancelled by the State Licensing Authority. Provided that, the renewal of a drug sale license shall be made before its expiry. However, if the licensee renews its license after expiry date within 6 months then, he needs to pay extra fees in the form of penalty fees every month which is applicable for 6 months only.

- Rule 63(A) - Certificate of renewal of a sale licence. The certificate of renewal of a sale licence in Forms 20, 20A, 20B, 20F, 20G, 21, 21A and 21B shall be issued in Form 21C.

  Interpretation -

  Rule 63(A) - The 'certificate of renewal' of a Retail Sale Drug License (Form 20, 21), Wholesale Drug License (Form 20B, 21B), Restrcited Drug Sale License (Form 20A, 21A), and Schedule X drug sale license (Form 20F, 20G) shall be issued in 'Form 21C'.

- Rule 63(B) - Certificate of renewal of licence. A certificate of renewal of a licence in Form 20BB or Form 21BB shall be issued in Form 21CC.
  Interpretation -
  Rule 63(B) - The 'certificate of renewal' of a motor vehicle drug sale license (Form 20BB and Form 21BB) shall be issued in Form 21CC.

- Rule 64 - Conditions to be satisfied before a licence in Form 20, 20B, 20F, 20G, 21 or 21B is granted.
  (1) A licence in Form 20, 20B, 20F, 20G, 21 or 21B to sell, stock, exhibit or offer for sale or distribute drugs shall not be granted, renewed to any person unless the authority empowered to grant the licence is satisfied that the premises in respect of which the licence is to be granted [or renewed] are adequate, equipped with proper storage accommodation for preserving the properties of the drugs to which the licence applies and are in charge of a person competent in the opinion of the licensing authority to supervise and control the sale, distribution and preservation of drugs : Provided that in the case of a pharmacy a licence in Form 20 or 21 shall not be granted or renewed unless the licensing authority is satisfied that the requirements prescribed for a pharmacy in Schedule N have been complied with: Provided further that licence in Form 20F shall be granted or renewed only to a pharmacy and in areas where a pharmacy is not operating, such licence may be granted or renewed to a chemist and druggist.
  Explanation. For the purpose of this rule the term 'Pharmacy' shall be held to mean to include every store or shop or other place :
  (1) where drugs are dispensed, that is, measured or weighed or made up and supplied ; or
  (2) where prescriptions are compounded; or
  (3) where drugs are prepared; or
  (4) which has upon it or displayed within it, or affixed to or used in connection with it, a sign bearing the word or words 'Pharmacy', 'Pharmacist', 'Dispensing Chemist' or 'Pharmaceutical Chemist'; or
  (5) which, by sign, symbol or indication within or upon it gives the impression that the operations mentioned at (1), (2) and (3) are carried out in the premises; or (6) which is advertised in terms referred to in (4) above.

  (2) In granting or renewing a licence under sub-rule (1) the authority empowered to grant it shall have regard -

(i) to the average number of licences granted or renewed during the period of 3 years immediately preceding, and

(ii) to the occupation, trade or business ordinarily carried on by such applicant during the period aforesaid.

Provided that the licensing authority may refuse to grant or renew a licence to any applicant or licensee in respect of whom it is satisfied that by reason of his conviction of an offence under the Act or these rules, or the previous cancellation or suspension of any licence granted or renewed thereunder, he is not a fit person to whom a licence should be granted or renewed under this rule. Every such order shall be communicated to the licensee as soon as possible:

Provided further that in respect of an application for the grant of a licence in Form 20B or Form 21B or both, the licensing authority shall satisfy himself that the premises in respect of which a wholesale licence is to be granted or renewed] are:-

(i) of an area of not less than ten square meters; and

(ii) in the charge of a competent person, who—

  (a) is a Registered Pharmacist, or

  (b) has passed the matriculation examination or its equivalent examination from a recognised Board with four years' experience in dealing with sale of drugs, or

  (c) holds a degree of a recognised University with one years experience in dealing with drugs.

Provided also that,-

(i) in respect of an application for the grant of a license in Form 20 or Form 21 or both, the licensing authority shall satisfy itself that the premises are of an area] of not less than 10 square meters, and

(ii) in respect of an application for the grant of a license

  (A) In Form 20 or Form 21 or both, and

  (B) In Form 20 B or Form 21B or both,

  the licensing authority shall satisfy itself that the premises are of an area not less than 15 square meters.

Provided also that the provisions of the preceding proviso shall not apply to the premises for which licences have been issued by the licensing authority before the commencement of the Drugs and Cosmetics (1st Amendment) Rules, 1997.

(3) Any person who is aggrieved by the order passed by the licensing authority in sub-Rule (1) may, within 30 days from the date of receipt of such order, appeal to the State Government and the State

Government may, after such enquiry into the matter as it considers necessary and after giving the appellant an opportunity for representing his views in the matter, make such an order in relation thereto as it thinks fit.

Interpretation -
Rule 64(1) - A drug sale license (for retail and wholesale drug license) in Form 20, 20B, 20F, 20G, 21 or 21B for stock, sale and distribution shall not be granted by the state licensing authority until and unless he is satisfied that, applicant's licensed premises are adequate, equipped with proper storage accommodation for preserving drug's properties and quality. Also, qualified person and person in-charge for licensed premise is competent enough to supervise and control the sale, distribution and preservation of drugs. Provided that, in the case of a 'pharmacy' a license in Form 20 or 21 (Retail sale drug license) shall not be granted or renewed unless the licensing authority is satisfied that the requirements prescribed for a 'pharmacy' prescribed under 'Schedule N' have been complied with. For Form 20F (Retail sale drug license for Schedule X Drugs) shall not be granted or renewed to a pharmacy where drug is being compounded, packed or made. Form 20F shall be only granted to 'Chemist and Druggist' where drug is only intended for dispensed by a endorsed registered pharmacist.

Explanation. For the purpose of this rule the term 'Pharmacy' shall be held to mean to include every store or shop or other place :
(1) where drugs are dispensed (giving medicine to a named person on the basis of a prescription), that is, measured or weighed or made up and supplied ; or
(2) where prescriptions are compounded (preparation, mixing, assembling, packaging or labeling of a drug or device as a result of a practitioner's prescription drug order); or
(3) where drugs are prepared; or
(4) which has upon it or displayed sign bearing the word or words 'Pharmacy', 'Pharmacist', 'Dispensing Chemist' or 'Pharmaceutical Chemist'; or
(5) which, by sign, symbol or indication where above operations mentioned at (1), (2) and (3) are carried out in the premises; or (6) which is advertised in terms referred to in (4) above.

Rule 64(2) - Regarding the license granted for a drug sale license (for retail and wholesale drug license) in Form 20, 20B, 20F, 20G, 21 or 21B for stock, sale and distribution, the State licesning authority shall have regard with respect to average number of licenses granted or renewed during the period of 3 years immediately preceding, and to the occupation, trade or business ordinarily carried on by such applicant during the period aforesaid.

Provided that, the state licensing authority may refuse to grant or renew a license to any applicant or licensee on the ground of applicant's previous conviction of an offence under the Act or these rules, or history of the previous license cancellation or suspension. Also, State licensing authority can refuse to grant or renew license if he finds that the applicant (person) is not a fit under this rule and every such order shall be communicated to the licensee as soon as possible for application rejection with reason.

Provided that, in case of grant of wholesale drug license (Form 20B, 21B) the state licensing authority shall satisfy himself that the premises for which wholesale drug license is to be granted or renewed should be:
(i) of an area of not less than 10 square meters; and
(ii) in the charge of a competent person, who is (a) Registered Pharmacist, or (b) Matriculation pass with 4 years experience in dealing with sale of drugs, or (c) graduate degree holder from a recognised University with 1 year experience in dealing with drugs.

Provided that,
(i) for grant of a 'retail sale drug license (Form 20, 21)' the area of the licensed premise shall be not less than 10 square meters (108 sq. ft.), and
(ii) for grant of a 'combined retail and wholesale drug license (i.e. Form 20, 21, 20B, 21B)' the area of the licensed premise shall be not less than 15 square meters (162 sq. ft.).

Provided that, above provisions and rules shall not apply to the licensed premises for which licences have been issued by the state licensing authority before the commencement of the Drugs and Cosmetics (1st Amendment) Rules, 1997.

Rule 64(3) - Any person who is aggrieved and not satisfied by the state licesning authority's order regarding rejection of grant or renewal of drug sale license in sub-Rule (1) may, within 30 days from the date of receipt of such order, can appeal to the State Government. On hearing plea filed by the appellant against license rejection order by the state licensing authority, the State Governement can give the appellant an opportunity for representing his views in the matter, and then make an order regarding this matter whichever he (State Governement) thinks fit.

- Rule 65 - Condition of licences (Licenses in Forms 20, 20A, 20B, 20F, 20G, 21, and 21B) shall be subject to the conditions stated therein and to the following general conditions.
Rule 65(1) - Any drug shall, if compounded or made on the licensee's premises be compounded or made by or under the direct and personal supervision of a Registered Pharmacist.

Interpretation -
Rule 65 - Condition of licenses for restricted sale drug license (Form 20A, 21A), retail sale drug license (Form 20, 21), wholesale drug license (Form 20B, 21B) and Schedule X drug sale license (Form 20F, 20G) shall be followed for the following general condition.
Rule 65(1) - Any drug shall, if 'compounded' (preparation, mixing, assembling, packaging or labeling of a drug or device) or 'made' inside the licensed premises or 'compounded/made' under the direct and personal supervision of a Registered Pharmacist only.

Rule 65(2) - The supply, otherwise than by way of wholesale dealing, of any drug supplied on the prescription of a Registered Medical Practitioner shall be effected only by or under the personal supervision of a registered Pharmacist.
Interpretation -
Rule 65(2) - The supply of any allopathic prescription drugs (except wholesale) against a prescription of a Registered Medical Practitioner (RMP) shall be carried out only under the personal supervision or physical presence of a Registered Pharmacist. The registered pharmacist's name shall be endorsed (mentioned) in the retail sale drug license (Form 20, 21).

Rule 65(3)(1) - The supply of any drug other than those specified in Schedule X on a prescription of a Registered Medical Practitioner shall be recorded at the time of supply in a prescription register specially maintained for the purpose and the serial number of the entry in the register shall be entered on the prescription. The following particulars shall be entered in the register:
(a) serial number of the entry,
(b) the date of supply,
(c) the name and address of the prescriber,
(d) the name and address of the patient, or the name and address of the owner of the animal if the drug supplied is for veterinary use,
(e) the name of the drug or preparation and the quantity or in the case of a medicine made up by the licensee, the ingredients and quantities thereof,
(f) in the case of a drug specified in Schedule C or Schedule H and Schedule H1 the name of the manufacturer of the drug, its batch number and the date of expiry of potency, if any,
(g) the signature of the registered Pharmacist by or under whose supervision the medicine was made up or supplied.
(h) the supply of a drug specified in Schedule H1 shall be recorded in a separate register at the time of the supply giving the name and address of the prescriber, the name of the patient, the name of the drug and the quantity supplied and such records shall be maintained for three years and be open for inspection.

Interpretation -
Rule 65(3)(1) - The supply of any drug (except Schedule X drugs) on a prescription of a Registered Medical Practitioner (RMP) shall be recorded at the time of supply in a 'Prescription Register (in modern times all these details are captured in the sales tax invoice). Also, the unique serial number shall be entered on the prescription for the track and trace of that particular prescription drug order with following details:
(a) Serial number ,
(b) Date of supply (date of drug sale),
(c) Name and address of the prescriber (Doctor/RMP),
(d) Name and address of the patient (in case of human drugs), or the name and address of the owner of the animal if the drug supplied is for veterinary use (in case of animal drugs),

(e) Name of the drug or preparation (Generic or Brand name) and, quantity or in the case of a medicine made up by the licensee, the ingredients and quantities thereof,

(f) In case of Schedule C or Schedule H and Schedule H1 the 'drug manufacturer's name', 'batch/lot number' and 'expiry date' if any,

(g) Signature of the endorsed Registered Pharmacist (whose name is mentioned in the drug sale license).

(h) Schedule H1 drug supply record or register shall be maintained including details - 'RMP's name', 'RMP's address', 'patient's name', 'drug name' and 'drug quantity supplied' to be maintained for three years and be open for inspection.

Provided that in the case of drugs which are not compounded in the premises and which are supplied from or in the original containers, the particulars specified in items (a) to (g) above may be entered in a cash or credit memo book, serially numbered and specially maintained for this purpose.

<u>Interpretation</u> - Provided that, if any drug is not compunded (combined, mixed, or ingredients alteration to create a medication tailored to the needs of an individual patient) in the drug licensed premise and are supplied in the original container (package) the details mentioned above from (a) to (g) have to be maintained by the licensee (in the form of modern day sale tax invoice). However, in modern times there are no medicines available which are compounded by a licensed pharmacy as the majority of the drugs comes in pre-packed forms by the manufacturer.

Provided further that if the medicine is supplied on a prescription on which the medicine has been supplied on a previous occasion and entries made in the prescription register, it shall be sufficient if the new entry in the register includes a serial number, the date of supply, the quantity supplied and a sufficient reference to an entry in the register recording the dispensing of the medicine on the previous occasion.

<u>Interpretation</u> - If any prescription medicines has been dispensed previously on same prescription then it is fine, if the new details in the tax sales invoice (prescription register) includes 'unique serial number', , 'date of supply' and 'supplied drug quantity' along with a previous dispensation reference number .

Provided also that it shall not be necessary to record the above details in the register or in the cash or credit memo particulars in respect of:
(i) any drugs supplied against prescription under the Employees State Insurance Scheme if all the above particulars are given in that prescription, and
(ii) any drug other than that specified in Schedule C or Schedule H and Schedule H1 if it is supplied in the original unopened container of the manufacturer and if the prescription is duly stamped at the time of supply with the name of the supplier and the date on which the supply was made and on condition that the provisions of sub-rule (4)(3) of this rule are complied with.

Interpretation - Provided that, in above case details mentioned from (a) to (g) as per the Rule 65(3)(1), it is not necessary to capture these details of the prescription on the tax sales invoice if -
1. These drugs are supplied against prescription under the Employees State Insurance (ESI) Scheme.
2. Schedule C, H and H1 drugs are supplied in the original unopened manufacturer's package with prescription duly stamped with supplier name, supply date and on the conditions of Rule 65(4)(3) are complied with.

Rule 65(3)(2) - The option to maintain a prescription register or a cash or credit memo book in respect of drugs and medicines which are supplied from or in the original container, shall be made in writing to the Licensing Authority at the time of application for the grant or renewal of the licence to sell by retail. Provided that the Licensing Authority may require records to be maintained only in prescription register if it is satisfied that the entries in the carbon copy of the cash or credit memo book are not legible.

Interpretation -
Rule 65(3)(2) - During time of application for the grant or renewal of a retail sale drug license (RSDL), the licensee shall provide all the details of dispensed prescription drugs maintained in the prescription register or cash/credit memo book (modern day tax sale invoice) to the State Licensing Authority (SLA). Provided that, SLA may require records to be maintained only in prescription register (modern day tax sale

invoice) in case duplicate copies or carbon copies of cash or credit memo book (modern day tax sale invoice) are not legible or not readable.

Rule 65(4)(1) - The supply by retail, otherwise than on a prescription of a drug specified in Schedule C shall be recorded at the time of supply either:
(i) in a register specially maintained for the purpose in which the following particulars shall be entered:
(a) serial number of the entry,
(b) the date of supply,
(c) the name and address of the purchaser,
(d) the name of the drug and the quantity thereof,
(e) in the case of a drug specified in Schedule C, the name of the manufacturer, the batch number and the date of expiry of potency,
(f) the signature of the person under whose supervision the sale was effected, **or**
(ii) in a cash or credit memo book, serially numbered containing all the particulars specified in items (b) to (f) of sub-clause (i) above.
NOTE: The entries in the carbon copy of the cash or credit memo which is retained by the licensee shall be maintained in a legible manner.

Interpretation -
Rule 65(4)(1) - A retail sale drug licensee except for Schedule C drugs shall maintain register/record at the time of supply either in:
Rule 65(4)(1)(i) - Register/Record shall be maintained by the licensee with following details:
(a) Invoice number/order id/special serial number
(b) Date of drug sale
(c) Purchaser i.e. Patient's name and address
(d) Drug name and quantity sold
(e) In case of Schedule C (manufacturer's name, batch/lot number and expiry date)
(f) signature of endorsed registered pharmacist (whose name is mentioned in the retail sale drug license).

Rule 65(4)(1)(ii) - The tax sales invoice shall be serially numbered containing all the details mentioned from (b) to (f) of sub-clause (i) above.

NOTE: The entries in the duplicate copies of the tax sale invoice (carbon copy of cash/credit memo) maintained by the retail sale drug licensee shall be in a legible manner or readable form.

Rule 65(4)(2) - The option to maintain a register or a cash or credit memo book shall be made in writing to the Licensing Authority at the time of application for the grant or renewal of a licence to sell by retail: Provided that the Licensing Authority may require records to be maintained in a register if it is satisfied that the entries in the carbon copy of the cash/credit memo book are not legible.

Interpretation -
Rule 65(4)(2) - The option to maintain a register or a cash or credit memo book (tax sale invoice) shall be made in writing and provided to the State Licensing Authority (SLA) during time of application for grant or renewal of a retail sale drug license (RSDL). In case carbon copy of cash/credit memo book (tax sale invoice) are not legible or readable, then SLA may ask to produce register with all records maintained by the retail sale drug licensee.

Rule 65(4)(3) -
(i) The supply by retail of any drug shall be made against a cash/credit memo which shall contain the following particulars :
    (a) Name, address and sale license number of the dealer,
    (b) Serial number of the cash/credit memo,
    (c) the name and quantity of the drug supplied.
(ii) Carbon copies of cash/credit memos shall be maintained by the licensee as record.

Interpretation -
Rule 65(4)(3)(i) - The supply of any drug by a **Retail** shall be made only against a cash/credit memo (modern day tax sale invoice) containing following details:
(a) Name, address and drug license number of the dealer (retailer),
(b) Serial number of the cash/credit memo (invoice number/order id),
(c) Name and quantity of the drug supplied.

Rule 65(4)(3)(ii) - Carbon copies of cash/credit memos (duplicate copies of tax sale invoice) shall be maintained by the retail sale drug licensee as record.

Rule 65(4)(4)(i) - Records of purchase of a drug intended for sale or sold by retail shall be maintained by the licensee and such records shall show the following particulars, namely:
- (a) the date of purchase,
- (b) the name and address of the person from whom purchased and the number of the relevant licence held by him,
- (c) the name of the drug, the quantity and the batch number, and
- (d) the name of the manufacturer of the drug.

(ii) Purchase bills including cash or credit memo shall be serially numbered by the licensee and maintained by him in a chronological order.

Interpretation -
Rule 65(4)(4)(i) - The purchase record (purchase tax invoice) of a drug intended for sale by **Retail** shall be maintained with following details:
- (a) Drug purchase date,
- (b) Name, address and drug license number of wholesaler/dealer or any entity from whom drug is purchased,
- (c) Drug name, quantity and batch/lot number, and
- (d) Drug manufacturer's name

Rule 65(4)(4)(ii) - Purchase invoices shall be serially numbered by the retail sale drug licensee and maintained by him in a chronological order (date wise manner).

Rule 65(5)(1) - Subject to the other provisions of these Rules the supply of a drug by wholesale shall be made against a cash or credit memo bearing the name and address of the licensee and his licence number under the Drugs and Cosmetics Act in which the following particulars shall be entered-
(a) the date of sale,
(b) the name, address of the licensee to whom sold and his sale licence number. In case of sale to an authority purchasing on behalf of Government, or to a hospital, medical, educational or research institution or to a Registered Medical Practitioner for the purpose of supply to his patients the name and address of the authority, institution or the Registered Medical Practitioner as the case may be,
(c) the name of the drug, the quantity and the batch number,
(d) the name of the manufacturer,

(e) the signature of the competent person under whose supervision the sale was effected.

Interpretation -
Rule 65(5)(1) - Supply of a drug by a **Wholesaler** shall be made only against a sales tax invoice bearing his name, address and wholesale drug license number with following details:
(a) Sale/supply date,
(b) Name, address, and drug license number of entity to whom sold. [*In case of wholesaler is selling drugs to 'authority purchasing on behalf of State or Central Government', or 'hospital' or 'medical educational' or 'research institution' or 'Qualified Allopathic Doctor/RMP for the purpose of supply to his patient' the name and address of the authority, institution or RMP (whichsoever)*],
(c) Drug name, quantity and batch/lot number,
(d) Manufacturer's name,
(e) Endorsed Competent Person (CP) whose name is mentioned in the wholesale drug license.

Rule 65(5)(2) - Carbon copies of cash or credit memos specified in clause (1) shall be preserved as records for a period of three years from the date of the sale of the drug.

Interpretation -
Rule 65(5)(2) - The duplicate copies of the purchase tax invoice shall be maintained by a wholesale drug licensee for a period of minimum 3 years from the date of sale of drug.

Rule 65(5)(3)(i) - Records of purchase of a drug intended for resale or sold by wholesale shall be maintained by the licensee and such records shall show the following particulars, namely:-
    (a) the date of purchase,
    (b) the name, address and the number of the relevant licence held by the person from whom purchased,
    (c) the name of the drug, the quantity and the batch number, and
    (d) the name of the manufacturer of the drug.
(ii) Purchase bills including cash or credit memos shall be serially numbered by the licensee and maintained by him in a chronological order.

Interpretation

Rule 65(5)(3)(i) - Records of purchase tax invoice of a drug intended for resale or sold by a **Wholesaler** shall be maintained with following details:
- (a) Drug purchase date,
- (b) Name, address and wholesale drug license number of entity from whom drug is purchased,
- (c) Drug name, quantity supplied and batch/lot number, and
- (d) Drug manufacturer name.

Rule 65(5)(3)(ii) - The purchase tax invoice of the drugs shall be serially numbered and maintained by the wholesale drug licensee in a chronological order (date wise manner).

Rule 65(6) - The licensee shall produce for inspection by an Inspector appointed under the Act on demand all registers and records maintained under these Rules, and shall supply to the Inspector such information as he may require for the purpose of ascertaining whether the provisions of the Act and Rules thereunder have been observed.

Interpretation -

Rule 65(6) - A Retailer or Wholesaler shall produce all the documents/records/registers as whenever required by a Drug Inspector during inspection related to the directors, owner, registered pharmacist, licensed premise, prescription register, drug pricing details, sales bill, purchase bills etc. prescribed under the Drugs and Cosmetics Act and Rules thereunder.

Rule 65(7) - Except where otherwise provided in these rules, all registers and records maintained under these rules shall be preserved for a period of not less than two years from the date of the last entry therein.

Interpretation -

Rule 65(7) - Except for rules provided in these rules, all the registers and records under the Drugs Rules shall be maintained for minimum 2 years from the date of last entry.

Rule 65(8) - Notwithstanding anything contained in this Rule it shall not be necessary to record particulars in a register specially maintained for the purpose if the particulars are recorded in any other register specially maintained under any other law for the time being in force.

Interpretation -
Rule 65(8) - It is not necessary to maintain all details in a register if details are recorded in any other register specially maintained under any other law for the time being in force. Example in the sales bill (sales tax invoice) all the details related to prescription, supplied drug and drug licensee, registered pharmacist/competent person signature are also captured. Hence, all details are getting captured at one place in the form of tax invoice/bill.

Rule 65(9)(a) - Substances specified in Schedule H, Schedule H1 or Schedule X shall not be sold by retail except on and in accordance with the prescription of a Registered Medical Practitioner and in the case of substances specified in Schedule X, the prescriptions shall be in duplicate, one copy of which shall be retained by the licensee for a period of two years.

Interpretation -
Rule 65(9)(a) - Allopathic prescription drugs (including Schedule H, H1 or X) shall not be sold by a Retailer to a patient or customer without a valid Doctor's prescription. In case of Schedule X drugs sold to a patient or customer a Retailer shall maintain a duplicate copy (photocopy) of a prescription for 2 years.

Rule 65(9)(b) - The supply of drugs specified in [Schedule H and Schedule H1] or Schedule X to Registered Medical Practitioners, Hospitals, Dispensaries and Nursing Homes shall be made only against the signed order in writing which shall be preserved by the licensee for a period of two years.

Interpretation -
Rule 65(9)(b) - In case a Retailer or Wholesaler is supplying Schedule H, H1 or X drugs to any Allopathic Doctor, Hospitals, Dispensaries and Nursing Homes then, it shall be made only against a signed order in writing to be maintained by licensee for min. 2 years.

Rule 65(10) - For the purposes of clause (9) a prescription shall-

(a) be in writing and be signed by the person giving it with his usual signature and be dated by him;
(b) specify the name and address of the person for whose treatment it is given, or the name and address of the owner of the animal if the drug is meant for veterinary use;
(c) indicate the total amount of the medicine to be supplied and the dose to be taken.

Interpretation -
Rule 65(10) - This Rule is applicable for prescription rule mentioned above in Drugs Rules 65(9) where a valid prescription shall contain the following details:
(a) Shall be in writing and contain the usual signature of the RMP with date.
(b) Name and address of patient (for human use drug) or, name and address of animal owner (for veterinary drug).
(c) Total amount/quantity and dose (medicine amount taken at any one time).

Rule 65(11) - The person dispensing a prescription containing a drug specified in Schedule H, Schedule H1 and Schedule X shall comply with the following requirements in addition to other requirements of these Rules -
(a) the prescription must not be dispensed more than once unless the prescriber has stated thereon that it may be dispensed more than once;
(b) if the prescription contains a direction that it may be dispensed a stated number of times or at stated intervals it must not be dispensed otherwise than in accordance with the directions;
(c) at the time of dispensing there must be noted on the prescription above the signature of the prescriber the name and address of the seller and the date on which the prescription is dispensed.

Interpretation -
Rule 65(11) - The endorsed Registered Pharmacist of a Retailer who is the authorized person to dispense the allopathic prescription drugs (including Schedule H, H1 and X drugs) to a patient or customer shall comply with the following compliance of the Drugs Rules:

(a) A Prescription must not be dispensed more than once. For a repeated dispensing of medicines on the same prescription, the RMP shall mention it on that same prescription that, it can be dispensed more than once.
(b) If a Prescription contains a direction by a RMP that, medicines can be dispensed twice, thrice etc. on the same prescription then, the same can be dispensed. In case, if no such RMP's direction is mentioned on the prescription then, it shall not be dispensed to the patient or customer.
(c) During medicine dispensing, name and address of the retail pharmacy (seller) along with the dispensing date shall be mentioned by the endorsed Registered Pharmacist on the prescription above the signature of the RMP.

Rule 65(11)(A) - No person dispensing a prescription containing substances specified in [Schedule H and Schedule H1] or X], may supply any other preparation, whether containing the same substance or not, in lieu thereof.

Interpretation -
Rule 65(11) - This implies that brand medicines substitution for allopathic drugs is not allowed and the endosred registered pharmacist shall dispense same branded drugs written on the RMP's prescription. However, if the RMP has clearly mentioned on the prescription that brand substitution is allowed but not without patient consent.

Rule 65(12) - Substances specified in Schedule X kept in retail shop or premises used in connection therewith shall be stored—
(a) under lock and key in cupboard or drawer reserved solely for the storage of these substances; or
(b) in a part of the premises separated from the remainder of the premises and to which only responsible persons have access.

Interpretation -
Rule 65(12) - Schedule X drugs, if sold by a Retailer on Form 20F and a Wholesaler on Form 20G shall be stored -
(a) Under a lock & key cupboard reserved for the purpose of storage of Schedule X drugs only.
(b) In the cupboard which shall be located separated from other drugs categories and to be accessed or opened by only the licensee's

responsible person like endorsed registered pharmacist only during dispensing.

Rule 65(15) -
 (a) The description 'Drugstore' shall be displayed by such licensees who do not require the services of a Registered Pharmacist.
 (b) The description 'Chemists and Druggists' shall be displayed by such licensees who employ the services of a Registered Pharmacist but who do not maintain a Pharmacy for compounding against prescriptions.
 (c) The description 'Pharmacy', 'Pharmacist', 'Dispensing Chemist' or 'Pharmaceutical Chemist' shall be displayed by such licensees who employ the services of a Registered Pharmacist and maintain a Pharmacy for compounding against prescriptions.

Explanation:- For the purpose of this rule,-
(i) Registered Pharmacist means a person who is a registered Pharmacist as defined in clause (i) of section (2) of the Pharmacy Act, 1948 (Act No. 8 of 1948): Provided that the provisions of sub-clause (i) shall not apply to those persons who are already approved as qualified personll by the licensing authority on or before 31st December, 1969.
(ii) Date of Expiry of potency means the date that is recorded on the container, label or wrapper as the date up to which the substance may be expected to retain a potency not less than or not to acquire a toxicity greater than that required or permitted by the prescribed test.

Interpretation -
Rule 65(15) -
The display board shall be displayed at the entry point with description word '<u>Drugstore</u>' by a retailer who do not employ services of a Registered Pharmacist (i.e. licensee who possess Form 20A and 21A).

The display board shall be displayed at the entry point with description word '<u>Chemists and Druggists</u>' by a retailer who employ the services of 'Registered Pharmacist' who do not compound drugs against prescription (i.e. combining, mixing, or altering ingredients to create a medication tailored to the needs of an individual patient). Usually under such license of 'Chemists and Druggists' the endorsed Registered Pharmacist dispense only the prepacked or prefabricated allopathic drugs to the patient against a prescription. This condition is applicable for a Retailer who possess Form 20, 21. When any licensee applies for such retail sale drug license then, the State Licensing Authority usually cut or omit the word *"and to operate a pharmacy"* in such license. Schedule N is also not applicable for this type of drug sale license.

The display board shall be displayed at the entry point with description word 'Pharmacy', 'Pharmacist', 'Dispensing Chemist' or 'Pharmaceutical Chemist' by a Retailer who employ the services of a 'Registered Pharmacist' involved in compounding (combining, mixing, or altering ingredients to create a medication tailored to the needs of an individual patient) drugs against a prescription. This condition is applicable for a retailer who possess Form 20, 21. When any licensee applies for such retail sale drug license then, standards and norms of Schedule N is applicable for them.

Explanation:- For the purpose of this rule,-
(i) 'Registered Pharmacist' means a person who is a registered Pharmacist as defined in the Section (2)(i) of Pharmacy Act, 1948 (8 of Pharmacy Act, 1948). Provided that Registered Pharmacist definition shall not apply to those persons who are already approved as qualified person by the licensing authority on or before 31st December, 1969.
(ii) 'Date of Expiry of potency' means the date that is mentioned on the drug label which substance i.e. drug's ingredients indicates the shelf life's final date that the manufacturer guarantees the full potency and safety of a medication.

Rule 65(16) - The licensee shall maintain an Inspection Book in Form 35 to enable an Inspector to record his impressions and the defects noticed.
Interpretation -
Rule 65(16) - A retailer or wholesaler shall maintain a 'Drug Inspector observational booklet' in Form 35 in the licensed premises which enables Drug Inspector to record his observations or impressions and the defects noticed. This Form 35 is available at the State Licesning Authority office from where a retailer or wholesaler can purchase the same.

Rule 65(17) - No drug shall be sold or stocked by the licensee after the date of expiration of potency recorded on its container, label or wrapper, or in violation of any statement or direction recorded on such container, label or wrapper: Provided that any such drugs in respect of which the licensee has taken steps with the manufacturer or his representative for the withdrawal, reimbursement or disposal of the same, may be stocked after the date of expiration of potency pending such withdrawal, reimbursement or disposal, as the case may be, subject to the condition that the same shall be stored separately from the trade stocks and all such drugs shall be kept in packages or cartons, the top of which shall display prominently, the words —Not for sale.

Interpretation -

Rule 65(17) - A retailer or wholesaler should not sell or stock any drugs which is 'Expired' or 'any violation regarding the statement or directions like storage conditions, warning etc. mentioned on the drug label. Provided that, for such expired drugs if a retailer or wholesaler has taken any steps with the manufacturer or his representative for the withdrawal, reimbursement or disposal may be stocked in the licensed premises on condition that, such expired drugs stocks shall be stored separately from the trade stocks in packages or cartons with word 'NOT FOR SALE' displayed on its top.

Rule 65(18) -

No drug intended for distribution to the medical profession as free sample which bears a label on the container as specified in clause 4 [(ix)] of sub-rule (1) of rule 96, and no drug meant for consumption by the Employees' State Insurance Corporation, the Central Government Health Scheme, the Government Medical Stores Depots, the Armed Forces Medical Stores or other Government institutions, which bears a distinguishing mark or any inscription on the drug or on the label affixed to the container thereof indicating this purpose shall be sold or stocked by the licensee on his premises:

Provided that this sub-rule shall not be applicable to licensees who have been appointed as approved chemists, by the State Government in writing, under the employees' State Insurance Scheme, or have been appointed as authorised agent or distributor, by the manufacturer in writing, for drugs meant for consumption under the Central Government Health Scheme, the Government Medical Stores Depots, the Armed Forces Medical Stores or other Government Institutions for drugs meant for consumption under those schemes or have been appointed as authorised Depots or Carrying and Forwarding agent by the manufacturer in writing, for storing free samples meant for distribution to medical profession subject to the conditions that the stock shall be stored separately from the trade stocks and shall maintain separate records of the stocks received and distributed by them.

Interpretation -

Rule 65(19) - No drug intended for 'distribution to Doctors as free sample' and 'meant for consumption by the Employees State Insurance Corporation (ESIC), Central Government Health Scheme, Government Medical Stores Depots, Armed Forces Medical Stores or other Government institutions, with inscription on its drug label indicating the purpose', shall be sold or stocked by the licensee in his licensed premise.

Provided that this Rule 65(17) shall not be applicable to licensees:

- Who have been appointed as Approved Chemists by the State Government in writing, under the employees' State Insurance Scheme, **or**
- Who have been appointed as authorized agent or distributor, by the manufacturer in writing, for drugs meant for consumption under the Central Government Health Scheme, the Government Medical Stores Depots, the Armed Forces Medical Stores or other Government Institutions for drugs meant for consumption under those schemes, **or**
- Who have been appointed as authorised Depots or Carrying and Forwarding Agent (CFA) by the manufacturer in writing.

For storing such free samples of the drugs meant for distribution to the Doctors on the conditions that, such stocks shall be stored separately from the trade stocks and shall maintain separate records of the stocks received and distributed by them.

Rule 65(19) - The supply by retail of any drug in a container other than the one in which the manufacturer has marketed the drug, shall be made only by dealers who employ the services of a Registered Pharmacist and such supply shall be made under the direct supervision of the Registered Pharmacist in an envelope or other suitable wrapper or container showing the following particulars on the label:

(a) name of the drug,
(b) the quantity supplied,
(c) the name and address of the dealer.

Interpretation -

Rule 65(18) - If a dealer/licensee supplies drugs in an envelope or wrapper or container of his own (other than manufacturer's original package) then he should ensure that:
- Dealer/Licensee should have a valid retail sale drug license.
- Dealer/Licensee should have employed a registered pharmacist.
- Dealer/Licensee should ensure that, all such supplies of drugs in licensee's own envelope, wrapper or container (package) other than manufacturer's package should show details on licensee' drug label which includes: name of drug, quantity of drug supplied/sold, name and address of dealer/licensee.

Rule 65(20) - The medicines for treatment of animals kept in a retail shop or premises shall be labelled with the words '*Not for human use - for treatment of animals only*' and shall be stored:
(a) in a cupboard or drawer reserved solely for the storage of veterinary drugs, or
(b) in a part of the premises separated from the remainder of the premises to which customers are not permitted to have access.
Interpretation -
Rule 65(20) - A retailer having a valid retail sale drug license shall label the veterinary drugs intended for use in animals with word '*Not for human use - for treatment of animals only*' and should be stored:
(a) In a cupboard or drawer or separate storage zone rack intended for storage of vetereninary drugs only.
(b) The veterinary drug storage area in the licensed premises should be separated from other drugs storage area where customer should not have direct entry access or be allowed to entered.

Rule 65 (21) -
(a) The supply of drugs specified in Schedule X shall be recorded at the time of supply in a register (bound and serially page numbered) specially maintained for the purpose and separate pages shall be allotted for each drug.
(b) The following particulars shall be entered in the said register, namely:-
 (i) Date of transaction;
 (ii) Quantity received, if any, the name and address of the supplier and the number of the relevant licence held by the supplier;
 (iii) Name of the drug;

(iv) Quantity supplied;
(v) Manufacturer's name;
(vi) Batch No. or Lot No;
(vii) Name and address of the patient/purchaser;
(viii) Reference Number of the prescription against which supplies were made;
(ix) Bill No and date in respect of purchases and supplies made by him;
(x) Signature of the person under whose supervision the drugs have been supplied.

Interpretation -
Rule 65(21) -
(a) The record of Schedule X drugs sold shall be recorded in a register (serially page numbered) specially maintained for the purpose and separate pages shall be allotted for each drug.
(b) The details of Schedule X drugs recodred in the register shall contains the following details:
(i) Date of transaction (supply or purchase).
(ii) Name, address and license number of the supplier or dealer from whom drug is purchased
(iii) Schedule X drug name;
(iv) Quantity supplied (sold);
(v) Manufacturer's name;
(vi) Batch No. or Lot No;
(vii) Name and address of the patient/purchaser;
(viii) Prescription reference number (modern day invoice number or Order ID) for the sold Schedule X drugs to patient;
(ix) Bill (Invoice) number with date of purchase or sale;
(x) Approved Qualified person's signature (under whose supervision the drugs have been supplied).

CHAPTER 10

New Law Reforms related to the Drugs and Pharmacy

1. **Jan Vishwas (Amendment of Provisions) Act, 2023:** This law was passed by the Ministry of Law and Justice (Legislative Department). It finally received the assent of the President and it is effective from 11th August, 2023. The main objective of the Act is to decriminalize minor offences that do not involve any harm to the public interest or national security and replace them with civil penalties or administrative actions. It also establishes a balance between the severity of the offence/violation committed and the gravity of the prescribed punishment.

Key features:
- Remove imprisonment clauses and/or fines in some provisions and convert them into penalties in some others.
- Introduces compounding of offences in some provisions, which means that the offenders can settle their cases by paying a certain amount without going through a court trial.
- Periodic revision of fines and penalties every 3 years, with an increase of 10% of the minimum amount for various offences in the specified Acts.

THE SCHEDULE
(See section 2)

SN	YEAR	NO.	SHORT TITLE	AMENDMENT
6	1940	23	The Drugs and Cosmetics Act, 1940	(A) In section 29, for the words "punishable with fine which may extend to five thousand rupees", the words "liable to penalty which may extend to one lakh rupees" shall be substituted.
				(B) In section 30, in sub-section (2), for the words "imprisonment which may extend to two years, or with fine which shall not be less than ten thousand rupees, or with both", the words "fine which shall not be less than five lakh rupees" shall be substituted.
				(C) In section 32B, in sub-section (1), after the words and figures "of section 13" the words, brackets, letters and figures "clause (d) of section 27 and clause (ii) of section 27A," shall be inserted.

(A) **Section 29 - Penalty for use of Government Analyst's report for advertising:** Whoever uses any report of a test or analysis made by the Central Drugs Laboratory or by a Government Analyst, or any extract from such report, for the purpose of advertising any drug or cosmetic, shall be <u>punishable with fine which may extend to five thousand rupees</u>.

Change in law - Whoever uses any report of a test or analysis made by the Central Drugs Laboratory or by a Government Analyst, or any extract from such report, for the purpose of advertising any drug or cosmetic, shall be <u>liable to penalty which may extend to one lakh rupees</u>.

(B) **Section 30 (2) - Penalty for subsequent offences:** Whoever, having been convicted of an offence under Section 29 is again convicted of an offence under the same section shall be punishable with <u>imprisonment which may extend to two years, or with fine which shall not be less than ten thousand rupees or with both</u>.

Change in law -Whoever, having been convicted of an offence under Section 29 is again convicted of an offence under the same section shall be punishable with <u>fine which shall not be less than five lakh rupees</u>.

(C) **Section 32 (B) - Compounding of certain offences:** (1) Notwithstanding anything contained in the Code of Criminal Procedure, 1973, (2 of 1974) any offence punishable under clause (b) of sub-section (1) <u>of section 13</u>, section 28 and section 28A of this Act (whether committed by a company or any officer thereof), not being an offence punishable with imprisonment only, or with imprisonment and also with fine, may, either before or after the institution of any prosecution, be compounded by the Central Government or by any State Government or any officer authorised in this behalf by the Central Government or a State Government, on payment for credit to that Government of such sum as that Government may, by rules made in this behalf, specify: Provided that such sum shall not, in any case, exceed the maximum amount of the fine which may be imposed under this Act for the offence so compounded: Provided further that in cases of subsequent offences, the same shall not be compoundable.

Change in law - Notwithstanding anything contained in the Code of Criminal Procedure, 1973, (2 of 1974) any offence punishable under clause (b) of sub-section (1) of section 13, <u>clause (d) of section 27 and clause (ii) of section 27A</u>, section 28 and section 28A of this Act (whether committed by a company or any officer thereof), not being an offence punishable with imprisonment only, or with imprisonment and also with fine, may, either before or after the institution of any prosecution, be compounded by the Central Government or by any State Government or any officer authorised in this behalf by the Central Government or a State Government, on payment for credit to that Government of such sum as that Government may, by rules made in this behalf, specify: Provided that such sum shall not, in any case, exceed the maximum amount of the fine which may be imposed under this Act for the offence so compounded: Provided further that in cases of subsequent offences, the same shall not be compoundable.

THE SCHEDULE
(See section 2)

SN	YEAR	NO.	SHORT TITLE	AMENDMENT
9	1948	8	The Pharmacy Act, 1948	(A) In section 18, in sub-section (2), after clause (h), the following clauses shall be inserted, namely:— "(i) the manner of holding inquiry and imposing penalty under sub-section (1) of section 43A; (j) the form and manner of preferring appeal under sub-section (2) of section 43A."
				(B) In section 26A, in sub-section (3), for the words "punishable with imprisonment for a term which may extend to six months, or with fine not exceeding one thousand rupees, or with both", the words "liable to penalty which may extend to one lakh rupees" shall be substituted.
				(C) In section 41, for sub-section (1), the following sub-

				section shall be substituted, namely:— "(1) If any person whose name is not for the time being entered in the register of the State falsely pretends that it is so entered or uses in connection with his name or title any words or letters reasonably calculated to suggest that his name is so entered, he shall be punishable on first conviction with fine which may extend to one lakh rupees and on subsequent conviction with imprisonment which may extend to three months or with fine not exceeding two lakh rupees, or with both: Provided that it shall be a defence if the name of the person is entered in the register of another State and that at the time of claim, an application for registration in the State had been made.".
				(D) In section 42, in sub-section (2), for the words "imprisonment for a term which may extend to six months, or with fine not exceeding one thousand rupees or with both", the words "imprisonment for a term which may extend to three months, or with fine which may extend to two lakh rupees, or with both" shall be substituted.

				(E) After section 43, the following section shall be inserted, namely:— "43A. Adjudication of penalties.— (1) For the purposes of adjudging the penalties under section 26A, the Central Government shall authorise the President of the State Council, where the alleged violation is committed, to be the adjudicating officer for holding an inquiry and impose penalty in the manner as may be prescribed under section 18, after giving any person concerned a reasonable opportunity of being heard. (2) Whoever is aggrieved by any order of the adjudicating officer may prefer an appeal to the President, Central Council, within a period of forty-five days from the date of receipt of such order in such form and manner as may be prescribed under section 18. (3) The President, Central Council may entertain an appeal after the expiry of forty-five days, if it is satisfied that the appellant was prevented from sufficient cause for filing the appeal within the said period. (4) No appeal shall be disposed of unless the appellant has been given a reasonable opportunity of being heard.

				(5) An appeal under sub-section (2) shall be disposed of within ninety days from the date of filing. (6) The amount of penalty imposed under sub-section (1), if not paid, may be recovered as an arrear of land revenue.".

(A) <u>Section 18 (2) - Power to make regulations</u>: (2) In particular and without prejudice to the generality of the foregoing power, such regulations may provide for-

(a) the management of the property of the Central Council;

(b) the manner in which elections under this Chapter shall be conducted;

(c) the summoning and holding of meetings of the Central Council, the times and places at which such meetings shall be held, the conduct of business thereat and the number of members necessary to constitute a quorum;

(d) the functions of the Executive Committee, the summoning and holding meetings thereof, the times and places at which such meetings shall be held, and the number of members necessary to constitute a quorum;

(e) the powers and duties of the President and Vice-President;

(f) the qualifications, the term of office and the powers and duties of the Registrar, Secretary, Inspectors and other officers and servants of the Central Council, including the amount and nature of the security to be furnished by the Registrar or any other officer or servant;

(g) the manner in which the Central Register shall be maintained and given publicity;

(h) constitution and functions of the committees other than Executive Committee, the summoning and holding of meetings thereof, the time and place at which such meetings shall be held, and the number of members necessary to constitute the quorum.

<u>Change in law</u> - In particular and without prejudice to the generality of the foregoing power, such regulations may provide for-

(a) the management of the property of the Central Council;

(b) the manner in which elections under this Chapter shall be conducted;

(c) the summoning and holding of meetings of the Central Council, the times and places at which such meetings shall be held, the conduct of business thereat and the number of members necessary to constitute a quorum;

(d) the functions of the Executive Committee, the summoning and holding meetings thereof, the times and places at which such meetings shall be held, and the number of members necessary to constitute a quorum;

(e) the powers and duties of the President and Vice-President;

(f) the qualifications, the term of office and the powers and duties of the Registrar, Secretary, Inspectors and other officers and servants of the Central Council, including the amount and nature of the security to be furnished by the Registrar or any other officer or servant;

(g) the manner in which the Central Register shall be maintained and given publicity;

(h) constitution and functions of the committees other than Executive Committee, the summoning and holding of meetings thereof, the time and place at which such meetings shall be held, and the number of members necessary to constitute the quorum;

(i) the manner of holding inquiry and imposing penalty under sub-section (1) of section 43A;

(j) the form and manner of preferring appeal under sub-section (2) of section 43A.

(B) Section 26 (A) (3) - Inspection: Any person wilfully obstructing an Inspector in the exercise of powers conferred on him by or under this Act or any rules made thereunder shall be punishable with imprisonment for a term which may extend to six months, or with fine not exceeding one thousand rupees, or with both.

Change in law - Any person wilfully obstructing an Inspector in the exercise of powers conferred on him by or under this Act or any rules made thereunder shall be liable to penalty which may extend to one lakh rupees.

(C) Section 41 (1) - Penalty for falsely claiming to be registered:
(1) If any person whose name is not for the time being entered in the register of the State falsely pretends that it is so entered or uses in connection with his name or title any words or letters reasonably calculated to suggest that his name is so entered, he shall be punishable on first conviction with fine

which may extend to five hundred rupees and on any subsequent conviction with imprisonment extending to six months or with fine not exceeding one thousand rupees or with both: Provided that it shall be a defence to show that the name of the accused is entered in the register of another State and that at the time of the alleged offence under this section an application for registration in the State had been made.

Change in law - (1) If any person whose name is not for the time being entered in the register of the State falsely pretends that it is so entered or uses in connection with his name or title any words or letters reasonably calculated to suggest that his name is so entered, he shall be punishable on first conviction with fine which may extend to one lakh rupees and on subsequent conviction with imprisonment which may extend to three months or with fine not exceeding two lakh rupees, or with both: Provided that it shall be a defence if the name of the person is entered in the register of another State and that at the time of claim, an application for registration in the State had been made.

(D) Section 42 (2) - Dispensing by unregistered persons: (2) Whoever contravenes the provisions of sub-section (1) shall be punishable with imprisonment for a term which may extend to six months, or with fine not exceeding one thousand rupees or with both.

Change in law - (2) Whoever contravenes the provisions of sub-section (1) shall be punishable with imprisonment for a term which may extend to three months, or with fine which may extend to two lakh rupees, or with both.

(E) Section 43 - Failure to surrender certificate of registration: After section 43, the following section shall be inserted, namely:— "43A. Adjudication of penalties.—

(1) For the purposes of adjudging the penalties under section 26A, the Central Government shall authorise the President of the State Council, where the alleged violation is committed, to be the adjudicating officer for holding an inquiry and impose penalty in the manner as may be prescribed under section 18, after giving any person concerned a reasonable opportunity of being heard.

(2) Whoever is aggrieved by any order of the adjudicating officer may prefer an appeal to the President, Central Council, within a period of forty-five days from the date of receipt of such order in such form and manner as may be prescribed under section 18.

(3) The President, Central Council may entertain an appeal after the expiry of forty-five days, if it is satisfied that the appellant was prevented from sufficient cause for filing the appeal within the said period.

(4) No appeal shall be disposed of unless the appellant has been given a reasonable opportunity of being heard.

(5) An appeal under sub-section (2) shall be disposed of within ninety days from the date of filing.

(6) The amount of penalty imposed under sub-section (1), if not paid, may be recovered as an arrear of land revenue.".

Change in law - Section 43 (A) - Adjudication of penalties:

(1) For the purposes of adjudging the penalties under section 26A, the Central Government shall authorise the President of the State Council, where the alleged violation is committed, to be the adjudicating officer for holding an inquiry and impose penalty in the manner as may be prescribed under section 18, after giving any person concerned a reasonable opportunity of being heard.

(2) Whoever is aggrieved by any order of the adjudicating officer may prefer an appeal to the President, Central Council, within a period of forty-five days from the date of receipt of such order in such form and manner as may be prescribed under section 18.

(3) The President, Central Council may entertain an appeal after the expiry of forty-five days, if it is satisfied that the appellant was prevented from sufficient cause for filing the appeal within the said period.

(4) No appeal shall be disposed of unless the appellant has been given a reasonable opportunity of being heard.

(5) An appeal under sub-section (2) shall be disposed of within ninety days from the date of filing.

(6) The amount of penalty imposed under sub-section (1), if not paid, may be recovered as an arrear of land revenue.

www.ingramcontent.com/pod-product-compliance
Ingram Content Group UK Ltd.
Pitfield, Milton Keynes, MK11 3LW, UK
UKHW020244240426
12048UKWH00026B/1605